SPORTS INJURIES AND ILLNESSES

Their Prevention and Treatment

SPORTS INJURIES AND ILLNESSES

Their Prevention and Treatment

Bob O'Connor, Ed.D.
Richard Budgett, M.B.B.S., M.A., Dip Sport Med.
Christine Wells, M.S., N.M.A.
Jerry Lewis, M.S., C.A.T.

The Crowood Press

Distributed by
Trafalgar Square
North Pomfret, Vermont 05053

First published in 1998 by
The Crowood Press Ltd
Ramsbury, Marlborough
Wiltshire SN8 2HR

British Library Cataloguing in Publication Data

A catalogue record for this book is available from the
British Library.

ISBN 1 86126 107 1

Typeset by Swindon Press Limited, Swindon, Wiltshire.

Printed and bound in Great Britain by
WBC Book Manufacturers, Mid Glamorgan

Contents

Foreword

This book is written for anyone exercising regularly or planning to start an exercise programme. The emphasis is on how to exercise effectively to improve your physical and mental health, as well as how to optimize your performance.

It covers the whole of sports and exercise medicine with sections on all the common sports injuries in a wide range of sports. Early recognition, effective first aid, and the best treatment and rehabilitation are all discussed. Immediate treatment of a sports injury can make all the difference to the speed and effectiveness of recovery. Once you've read this book you will know what to do immediately and when to seek help.

It also gives lots of useful advice on the prevention of injury and illness, from common sprains to the overtraining syndrome. This is done through diet, cross training and conditioning. I hope you will enjoy and benefit from exercise while minimizing the risk of injury and illness, and that this book will help you do that.

Steve Redgrave C.B.E.
Four times Olympic Gold Medallist

Introduction

Physical fitness is an essential part of a healthy life. Adequate exercise not only makes us feel good but makes us look better, while controlling our weight and minimizing our risk of many diseases. The risk of having a heart attack, contracting some cancers, and diabetes, and even suffering from the common cold can be greatly reduced.

Although exercise is undoubtedly good for us, there can be the occasional downside to any physical activity. A sprained ankle, a bruise, blisters, or even a broken bone – all are a real possibility. Additionally, it is now known that exercise can even create some negative by-products in the body that must be neutralized if we are to live longer and better.

Just as there are physical benefits and physical problems, there are mental benefits and there can be mental problems. Effective exercise lowers our depression levels and makes us feel more positive about living. It also reduces the stresses that come from other areas of our life. However, too much exercise, a condition called 'over-training', can increase some harmful hormones and make us feel depressed. Fortunately, most active people never reach that state of over-training and staleness.

This book has two main focuses. The first is the care and treatment of common athletic injuries. The second is the prevention of injuries and other problems through proper nutrition, strength training, and the awareness of some problems that may occur with those who exercise and train at a very high level.

Exercise and sport can lead to better health. There are two main types of exercise – aerobic and strength. Aerobic exercise makes your heart beat fast for at least 20 to 30 minutes. It has the following benefits:

1. increasing the red blood cells that carry oxygen to the tissues. With more red cells, the heart does not have to work as hard to bring sufficient oxygen to the muscles and other tissues, having more rest time between beats;
2. increasing the capacity of the heart so that fewer beats per minute are required for the heart to do its necessary work;
3. increasing many of the white cells and other immunity factors which can reduce the rate of infection and the development of some cancers;
4. reducing the risk of, or the effects of, diabetes;
5. keeping the body physiologically younger;
6. reducing the chance of being over-weight;
7. reducing harmful blood fats, which can increase the likelihood of heart disease.

Strength exercise has the following benefits:
1. firms the muscles;
2. strengthens the bones.

Injuries are a fact of life. The English Sports Council recently found that there were 19.3

million sports injuries in a year in England and Wales. Of these injuries, 8.6 million were the result of involvement in soccer.

Finding the right practitioner – physician or medical person – is sometimes a challenge. You should be aware that not every trained therapist is qualified to work effectively with all sports injuries.

In this book we have attempted to bring you the latest in the medical sciences relating to the prevention and treatment of the injuries and other problems which often accompany athletic training and competition. Most people are aware of both the joys and the physical benefits that accrue from sport participation. Many are also aware that there are times when all doesn't go as well as it should. Our aim is to alert you to how you can prevent problems, but also to enable you both to recognize and to treat a problem if it does occur.

We hope that you enjoy reading the book as much as we have enjoyed writing it.

CHAPTER 1
Understanding and Treating Your Injuries

THE STRUCTURE OF THE BODY

In order to understand athletic injuries, it is essential to have some knowledge of the make-up of body structures and how they help you perform and function properly.

The major building block of the body is the *skeletal system* shown in Figs 1–3. The bones are quite different from each other in their construction and function. The longer bones of the arms, legs, hands and feet have a hollow shaft over which there is a covering on the bone and the bone material itself. Inside the hollow area are cells that produce the red blood cells, which carry oxygen, and white blood cells, which fight infection. Towards the ends of the bones, there are areas that allow growth in children and ado-

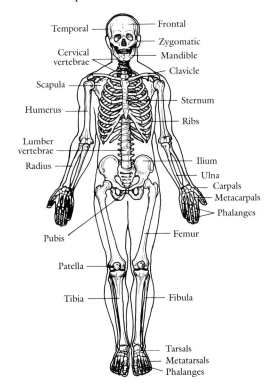

Fig 1. Front view.

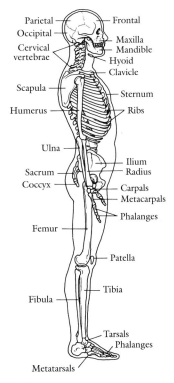

Fig 2. Side view.

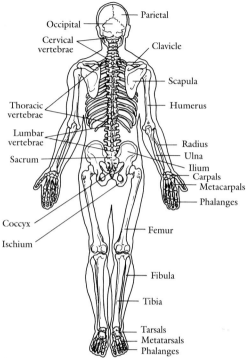

Fig 3. Rear view.

lescents. These are called growth plates. Many injuries to bones occur at the growth plates, since the growth plates are very soft and have immature cells. When tendons (which attach the muscles to the bones) or ligaments (which connect one bone to another) are attached to the growth plates, the growth plates can be pulled out of the bone.

A *joint* is where two bone ends come together. A joint is significant in that it allows two bones to move or articulate in a particular way, allowing the athlete to perform. The joint is surrounded by a membrane called the *joint capsule*. The joint capsule helps to hold fluid in the joint area.

At the ends of the bones is a material called *cartilage*. This material is softer than the bone and is very smooth. It allows the bones to slide past each other, or the tops of the bones that are touching each other to move with little friction. This is aided by the

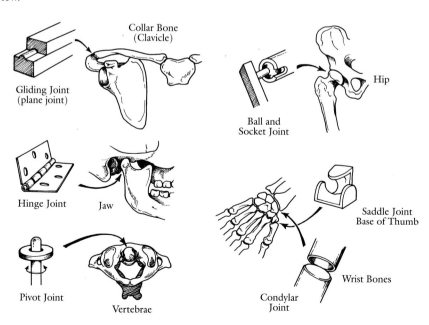

Fig 4

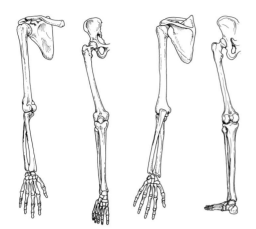

Fig 5. Comparison of arm and leg bones.

lubricating fluid that is contained in the joint capsule.

Joints have different functions. For example, a finger joint is designed to allow the finger to flex inwards but not outwards. A shoulder joint, on the other hand, allows the upper arm bone *(humerus)* to move in any direction and to twist, and it is, therefore, inherently less stable than the finger joint.

The movement of the bones at the joint can be reduced if the *ligaments* in the area are tight. Ligaments attach bone to bone. When a ligament is over-stretched it is called a sprain.

The ligament at the outside of the ankle is designed to stop the foot from turning

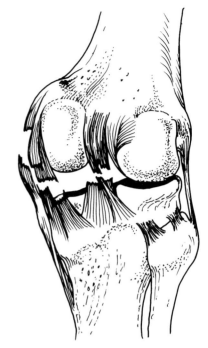

Fig 7. Torn knee ligaments.

inwards too far. Most ankle sprains cause damage to this ligament, and, being stretched, the ligament cannot do an effective job in holding the outside of the foot up. Some ligaments help to keep the bones close together, and prevent the joint making movements that would be detrimental to it when in use.

A *dislocation* occurs when ligaments are severely stretched and the bones of the joint move far from their normal alignment. Dislocated ankles, shoulders and elbows are not uncommon as sports injuries, particularly in contact sports. Shoulder dislocations are common when a sportsperson falls and attempts to cushion the fall with a straight arm.

The bones are moved by the *muscles*. The muscles are attached to the bones by *tendons*. The tendon is generally attached to an area of the bone that will give the best

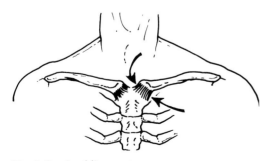

Fig 6. Sprained ligament.

mechanical leverage possible, so that a force may be applied to an outside object away from the body, or the body may be made to move in a specific way. For example, if the tendon that holds the bicep muscle to the lower arm were to be moved to half-way between where it is and the elbow joint, the strength of the arm would be reduced by 75 per cent.

The tendons attach into the bones at one end and into the muscle at the other. Muscle tissue is very elastic and the muscle cells are quite different from tendon cells. The point where the tendon and the muscle connect (the *muscle–tendon junction*) is an area of common injury. Awareness of this type of injury is very useful.

It is also important to be aware of the area where a muscle covers a joint, the area where a tendon goes across a joint, or the area where one bone is on top of another. Where the bone moves over that joint there is a small structure called a *bursa* – a sac or a sac-like cavity that contains fluid to help to cushion and lubricate the area. There is a large bursa in the shoulder to protect the deltoid muscle (going over the top of the shoulder joint) from being rubbed over the top of the humerus, so that the deltoid will not be torn by the humerus bone. In the knee, more than one bursa helps the knee joint to work. They are both above and below the tendons, above and below the bones, and above and below the muscles. They allow proper movement of the knee, and prevent problems that might be caused by these structures rubbing on top of each other.

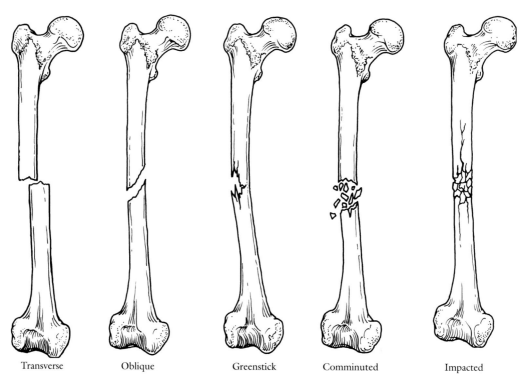

| Transverse | Oblique | Greenstick | Comminuted | Impacted |

Fig 8. Fracture types.

Quite often, because of over-use or out-side trauma, the bursa may be irritated or injured. When this occurs, the blood vessels feeding the bursa become damaged and the bursa swells and accumulates more fluid. The bursa can expand to up to five times its normal size. This inflammation of the bursa is called *bursitis,* occurs most often in the knee, shoulder or elbow, and shows itself by a bulging of the area. The bursa's swelling protects the structures around it.

A *trauma* to a bone may be one of a number of different types. *Fractures* are many and varied, and the simple break with which we are all familiar is just one type. A fracture may be *spiral* (up and down the shaft), *straight* across the shaft, or *angular,* diagonally across the shaft. It may be a clean break, or only a part of the bone may be broken. A *compression fracture* may be many small breaks in one area. For a discussion of the simple fracture, see the first-aid section (page 83).

WHAT HAPPENS WHEN A BODY IS INJURED?

When there is an injury, *bruising* usually occurs. A bruise is a breakage of the blood vessels, usually the small blood vessels *(capillaries)*. The initial reddish colour of the skin occurs because the blood in the capillaries is red, having just come through the arteries from the heart and lungs where it absorbed oxygen. As the oxygen in the blood is used by the tissues near the bruise, the blood becomes a darker red. As the oxygen is used, it appears blue in the veins that are going back to the heart. This soon gives the bruise the black and blue colour so characteristic of older bruises. A black eye is one of these older bruises.

When there is bleeding a *blood clot* forms. Just as a scab develops on the outside of the skin, a blood clot forms on the inside of a bruised muscle.

Scar tissue begins forming as a wound heals. While the normal body cells grow in an orderly way, scar tissue develops without any order, growing in all directions. When the injured area is stretched after scarring has occurred, the scar tissues that are in line with the normal tissues will stay intact, but the ones that are not in line with normal tissues will be stretched and torn with each movement. This will be painful, and happens whether the injury is in the skin tissue, a tendon, a ligament, or a joint capsule. The tissue will be torn when the sporting activity is taken up again. Normally, healing creates three to five times as much scar tissue as is needed.

Standard Treatment for Injuries

The purpose of standard treatment is to stop swelling and stop scar tissue from developing. The first measure of standard treatment is to apply some type of pressure, using an

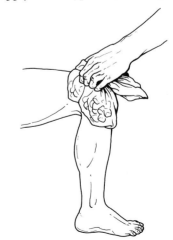

Fig 9. Apply ice bag to knee injury.

elastic bandage or by taping the area, for example.

Where specific advice on 'What to do' for each injury is given, the initials *R.I.C.E.* are often used. This is an acronym for *Rest, Ice, Compression,* and *Elevation.* Most injuries require this R.I.C.E. treatment, which is designed to reduce swelling, but healing the injury generally requires additional treatment. Below are the more complete standard treatments for injuries – measures which are commonly taken by those who treat athletic injuries professionally.

The 'standard treatment' will help pulled muscles, twisted knees, twisted or sprained ankles, elbow problems, shoulder injuries, and low back pain due to injury. It will not help a broken arm, which will not heal any sooner than 4-6 weeks, and needs immediate medical attention.

Phase 1: The First Three Days

The goal is to stop and reduce swelling by completely enclosing the whole injured area in ice or iced water. The coldness will reduce the blood circulation and thereby reduce swelling and scarring. A sprained ankle could be put into a bucket filled with iced water, but a knee would need a larger enclosure, such as a bath. The water should be at 55-60 degrees Fahrenheit (13-15 degrees centigrade). The length of time that each body part needs in cold water or ice may vary. For example, it has been found that using ice on a knee for twenty-five minutes is four times more effective in decreasing the blood flow to the knee than icing it for five minutes.

Apply the ice or iced water for twenty minutes every two hours and, if necessary, continue this treatment for seventy-two hours. If, after twenty-four hours, the swelling has gone down, or remained the same, the next step in the treatment would be to begin heat, which promotes healing. If the swelling is stopped in the first twenty-four to seventy-two hours, continuing to apply cold to the area is acceptable, but it delays the opportunity to begin healing by the proper use of heat.

The body usually gets rid of much of the swelling before it begins to heal. If there is a lot of swelling, the body will take longer to begin the healing process in the area of the injury. The goal is to stop the swelling as much as possible before adding the heat that will help to heal the injury.

Phase 2: The Second Three Days

This time should be used both to reduce swelling and to promote healing. It is best to submerge the injured area in hot water, but heat retainers can also be used. While the injured area is in the hot water, the blood vessels are opening, bringing all the nutrients and enzymes into the area and beginning the healing process. Heat should be about 105-110 degrees Fahrenheit (41-44 degrees centigrade). It should not be applied for too long.

The standard treatment in the second 72-hour period would be: one minute hot, three minutes cold, alternating five times, ending with five minutes of ice, to shut down any blood vessels that may have opened due to the heat and begun bleeding again.

Phase 3: The Third Three-Day Period

This period emphasizes increased healing by more use of heat. During this period of treatment, subtract one minute from the cold-water time and add that minute to the hot-water time – two minutes in the hot water, two minutes in the cold. Alternate this treatment five times, ending with five minutes of cold to shut down the blood vessels that are still not completely healed.

This should be done two to five times a day, if it is possible to fit this in with the normal daily routine. Treat the injury once before going to the office or to school, and give it another treatment if you have a break mid-morning. You may need to use hot packs (which can be heated in a small pan of water) and cold packs (ice cubes or a pack which can be put in the freezer) at this time. Lunch-time is another opportunity for a treatment. Repeat after school or work and before beginning any exercise. Do not repeat the treatment immediately after exercise, but use ice or iced water to reduce any swelling. The last treatment of hot and cold should be just before bedtime. Following this schedule gives five treatments a day, even during a busy day.

The more frequently the hot and cold treatment is done, the more the healing process is accelerated. This hot and cold treatment is done for seventy-two hours.

Phase 4: The Fourth Three-Day Period

Use three minutes hot, one minute cold, alternating five times, ending with five minutes of cold five times a day. At the end of the fourth 72-hour period, which is twelve days, the treatment is ten minutes of hot treatment four to five times a day. Do not try to accelerate the treatment by using more than ten minutes, as this is likely to cause more problems, such as unwanted swelling.

If any swelling is noticed, go back to cutting down on heat and add more cold to control the swelling. If necessary, go all the way back to one minute of hot and three minutes of cold, and work back up again.

After twenty-four days, the injured part of the body should be nearly back to normal. It may be possible to proceed more quickly through the phases if the injured person is well conditioned, because the circulatory system is usually more efficient, bringing the enzymes and nutrients to the injury quickly and continuously. Often, heat may be started almost immediately, possibly within twenty-four hours of the injury. On the other hand, if it is early in the training season, or the injured person is in poor physical condition, the treatment phases will have to be treated as three-day periods.

Standard treatment for any injury, except a full muscle or tendon tear, dislocation or fracture:

First 3 days: icing for 20 minutes every 2 hours.
(If a joint injury, begin manipulating the joint during the cold treatment.)

Second three days: 1 minute hot, 3 minutes cold.

Third three days: 2 minutes hot, 2 minutes cold.

Fourth three days: 3 minutes hot, 1 minute cold.

Thereafter: 10 minutes hot.

When no swelling, increase heat to 20 minutes per session.

Standard treatment and rehabilitation principles apply for each joint. Keep the swelling down and break up the scar tissue. Remember that when the scar tissue is being broken down, swelling may occur.

Always be aware of the possibility of more serious injury. If good progress is not made, see a properly qualified professional such as a doctor or chartered physiotherapist, who is ideally a sports medicine specialist.

Additional Therapy

Additional therapy during this time will include exercises. These should be begun as soon as possible after the injury. The earlier exercises are begun, the less scar tissue will be formed. While the injured area, particularly a joint, is being iced, make sure it is taken through a full range of movements.

Below is a programme of movement for a sprained ankle.
1. Check the range of motion, to see how far the ankle can be moved in every direction;
2. take the ball of the foot and press the foot upwards; this is called *flexing,* or *dorsiflexion;*
3. move the foot downwards; this is called *extension* or *plantar flexion;*
4. move the foot inwards, so that the sole of the foot is facing towards the other foot – *inversion;*
5. roll the foot outwards so that the sole is facing away from the other foot – *eversion.*

During the first seventy-two hours these movements should be done ten times during the icing phase of your treatment. In the second 72-hour period, while doing three minutes of ice, move the joint a great deal.

Because the ice is shutting down the blood vessels, swelling can be controlled.

Protecting the Injured Area

Protecting an injured area is important if the injured person plans to continue taking part in sport while the injury heals. When an injury is to soft tissue, such as the skin or a muscle, a doughnut-shaped pad is used to keep pressure off the injury and distribute it to the surrounding tissue. Injuries from blisters to large muscle bruises can be protected. Depending on the size of the injury, an appropriately thick pad should be used. For a small blister, a few thicknesses of gauze pads will do. To protect a larger area, a thick felt or heavy sponge rubber 'doughnut' will work. Athletic training suppliers usually have round- or oval-shaped pads specifically made for such protection. This will then be covered with a thicker pad that protects the injury and directs the weight to the underlying 'doughnut'. Protected in this way, the injury will not be further irritated.

Commonly Used Terms

Abduction: to take a body part away from the mid-line of the body, for example, raising the arm to the side.

Acute: a sudden problem.

Adduction: to bring a body part back to the body, for example, bringing a raised arm back to the side of the body.

Avulsion fracture: a break in the bone caused by a ligament or tendon pulling off a bone chip where it is attached.

Bursa: a sac of fluid that provides cushioning and protection around a joint.

Cartilage: a fibrous type of connective tissue. Some cartilage will become bone as the body ages.

Compression: putting pressure on a body part, for example, with an elastic bandage.

Concentric contraction: a muscular contraction during which the muscle is shortening, as when lifting a cup of coffee or lifting a weight over the head.

Connective tissue: a tough tissue that connects bone to bone (ligament), muscle to bone (tendon), or muscle to muscle.

Contusion: a blow to the soft tissue, such as a muscle, which causes bleeding, and a bruise.

Chronic: a long-standing problem.

Disc: a cartilage-like soft-centred pad that rests between each vertebra and helps to absorb the shocks which the back must endure.

Dislocation: the movement of a bone out of its normal position in a joint.

Eccentric contraction: a muscular contraction during which the muscle is lengthening (stretched), as when bending forward from a standing position, when the muscles of the back are lengthening.

Eversion: turning inwards.

Extension: opening up the angle of a joint and returning the body part to the straightened position from a flexed position, as when straightening the arm or leg, or bringing the torso upwards from a bent forward position.

Fascia: a sheet or band of connective tissue.

Flexion: bending a part of the body away from the normal standing position, as when bending the torso forward, bringing the hand closer to the shoulder, or bringing the foot closer to the hip by bending at the knee.

Fracture: a breaking of a bone, caused by a single trauma or by continued stresses *(stress fracture)*. *See also* Avulsion fracture.

Hyper-extension: going past the normal extended position, as when bending backwards, or bringing the fingers or toes up past their straightened position.

Inversion: turning inwards.

Isometric contraction: a muscular contraction in which the joint does not move, as when standing without moving.

Ligament: a type of tough connective tissue which holds one bone to another.

Muscle: an organ that includes contractile tissues that move the joints of the body when it contracts.

NSAIDs: non-steroidal anti-inflammatory drugs such as aspirin and ibuprofen.

Plyometrics: exercises that use the stretch-shortening cycle, such as repeated bounding jumps.

Prone: face down, lying on the front, or the palm of the hand held down.

Pronation: moving the body part to a prone position.

R.I.C.E.: shorthand for the essentials of treating most injuries – Rest, Ice, Compression, Elevation.

Spasm: a sudden and involuntary muscle contraction, such as a cramp.

Sprain: a stretching of a ligament. It can be mild, as in a simple stretching, or severe, in which the ligament is torn.

Strain: a stretching injury of a muscle or a tendon that attaches the muscle to a bone.

Stretch-shortening cycle: the action within a muscle in which it is stretched then shortened quickly. Jumping off a chair and immediately jumping upwards is such an action, as is striding forwards then pushing backwards with the leg.

Subluxation: a partial dislocation.

Supination: moving to a supine position.

Supine: facing up, lying on the back, or the hand held palm up, like a waiter carrying a tray.

Tendon: a type of connective tissue that connects muscle to bone.

Vertebra: one of the bones in the spinal column, protecting the spinal cord.

CHAPTER 2
The Foot

STRUCTURE

The foot is made up of approximately twenty-five bones. The heel bone is called the *calcaneus;* sitting on top of that is the *talus* bone, which goes up into the ankle to make part of the ankle joint. There are five bones in the front of the ankle, called the *tarsals.* In front of these are the five long foot bones going towards the toes, called the *metatarsals.* The first metatarsal is on the big toe side and the fifth metatarsal is on the little toe side. The toe bones are called the *phalanges.*

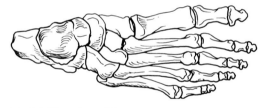

Fig 10. Top view of foot.

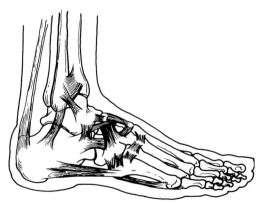

Fig 11. Outside view of ankle ligament.

The bones are held in two arches that go both from the toe to the heel and from the big toe to the little toe. These arches act as shock absorbers when walking, running or jumping. The arch involved in most athletic injuries is the longitudinal arch that goes from the ball of the foot back to the heel bone.

The bones are held together by ligaments at the joints; in every place where two bone ends come together there are ligaments. A joint capsule surrounds the joint to hold in fluid that allows the bone ends to move easily against one another. This gives the foot the flexibility needed to perform the movements that help to propel the body, and also to absorb and cushion the shock of walking, running and jumping activities.

SOFT-TISSUE INJURIES

The most common injuries to the foot are soft-tissue injuries, and the most common of these are blisters and calluses.

Blisters

Blisters are caused by rubbing of the skin, when the outer layer separates from the inner layer. When too much friction is put on the skin, it heats the skin and causes irritation and tissue damage, and a blister. The first and second layers separate and the fluid from the second layer fills that separation. The more friction and the more heat produced, the larger the blister. The fluid inside the blister causes pain.

Blisters are most common on the back of the heel, on the toes, or under the ball of the foot. Stiff-heeled shoes, shoes not properly laced, shoes that are too big or too small, and new sports shoes can all cause a blister. Blisters are far more likely at the beginning of a sports season, and football, basketball and running are the most likely sports in which early-season blisters will occur.

The blister should be treated quickly to reduce the amount of damage done. A trained medical person may disinfect the area, slit the side of the blister and pack it with a sterile gel. This can allow the athlete immediately to continue the event, but it should not be done by an untrained person. The danger of infection is too high.

What to do:
1. use a doughnut-shaped pad around the blister to eliminate any more pressure;
2. use a skin lubricant such as Vaseline over the blister, to protect it from any additional stress;
3. keep the area clean; the blister may pop on its own and infection must be avoided.

To prevent blisters:
1. file down any calluses so that blisters do not develop under them;
2. always wear socks when you are wearing shoes;
3. buy shoes with a proper fit and break in new shoes gradually;
4. *never* buy shoes by mail order; always try them on first.

A trained medical person would puncture a blister as follows: the skin is sterilized with alcohol or another antiseptic; a well-steril-ized needle is pushed through the first layer of skin of the blister and the fluid drained. The blister should *not* be popped open or ripped or cut open. The hole created should be small enough to heal itself quickly, to minimize the chance of infection. If the blister is allowed to continue swelling and filling with fluid from the second layer of skin, draining the blister with a needle would need to be repeated.

Calluses

If the skin is continually irritated in the manner that causes blisters, the third layer of skin becomes stimulated and more cells are produced to make the skin thicker. The more the growth rate is accelerated, the thicker the skin becomes, and the third layer of skin, the dead part seen on the outside, gets thicker and thicker and becomes what is called a *callus*.

If a callus is allowed to get too thick, too hard and too dried out, it becomes a source of irritation to the skin below, and a blister will form under it. In this way, a vicious cycle is begun. Calluses should be trimmed, filed, cut or treated so that the thickness of the callus will not continue to cause blisters to form underneath.

If the blisters continue to form and the calluses continue to grow, the skin must be protected from the pressure or friction by padding around that area with a doughnut-like pad. Cut a hole the same size as the blister, in the middle of a protective material, such as a gauze pad, thick felt or sponge rubber. Place this around the blister, and put some type of lubricant such as Vaseline inside the hole. Put another thin layer of gauze on top of it and tape it down. When there is pressure on the upper layer of gauze pad, it will be distributed out and around the blister on to the padding surrounding the blister, and the blister will be touched only by the lubricant.

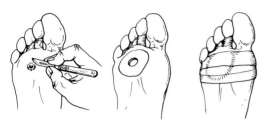

Fig 12. Blister treatment.

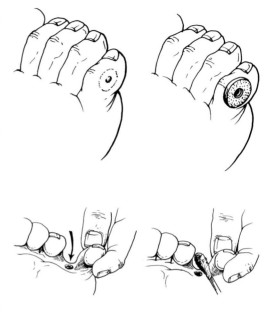

Fig 13. Corns.

Corns

Soft corns and hard corns may also develop, particularly on the top of the toes (usually hard corns), and in between the toes (usually soft). Corns are similar to calluses. They are also caused by pressure from the shoes, with the toes being squeezed tightly.

The pressure needs to be relieved. If the corn is a soft corn between the toes, put padding between toes. Widen the shoes or buy wider and longer shoes so that the pressure is relieved. The soft corns usually have a white scaly look about them and are moist and need to be dried out. The hard corns need to have a doughnut-shaped pad on top of them.

Bunions

Bunions are increased angles inwards of the big toe. The tendon on top of the toe pulls like a bowstring, making the angle worse. This causes the big toe joint to stick out further inwards, and a sore callus can develop here from pressure on the side of the shoe.

What to do:
1. wear a pad between the first and second toes to straighten the joint and reduce the pressure from the side;
2. wear a wider shoe to accommodate the inflamed bunion and the movement outward of the big toe joint;
3. R.I.C.E. especially after exercise. Do not use heat because it will increase the inflammation.

Verrucas

Plantar warts, or verrucas, are another type of soft-tissue problem, caused by a viral infection that can be irritated by pressure. They have a small core or kernel in the middle that may be dark and/or spread out. They also have roots growing into the skin tissue, trying to get nourishment from the third layer of skin where the capillaries are located. If pressure on the bottom of the foot is not relieved, the plantar warts will continue to grow until they become hard kernels that will cause pain with each step. Plantar warts are most likely to occur underneath the big toe, on the ball of the foot, or under the little toe where it connects to the foot; they sometimes appear on the outside of the heel, or directly on the bottom of the heel.

A doughnut-shaped pad will give relief by getting rid of the pressure that irritates plantar warts. An ill-fitting shoe is often the culprit, and wearing sandals can greatly reduce the pressure.

What to do:
1. use wart paint or see a doctor for further treatment;
2. form pads, or buy special pads, which will protect the wart from pressure.

THE HEEL

Stone Bruises

A bruised heel happens particularly frequently when sportspeople go barefoot or wear thin-heeled shoes and step accidentally on a stone. It also occurs with runners and jumpers who continually land on the base of the heel rather than on the toes. The pain may be quite sharp and may feel like a stone in the heel of the shoe.

What to do:
1. use R.I.C.E. for twenty to thirty minutes after exercise;

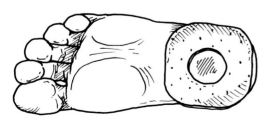

Fig 14. Heel doughnut.

2. massage the bottom of the heel with an ice cup (a cup of water placed in the freezer);
3. use a soft rubber heel cup or a doughnut-shaped felt pad with the hole in the doughnut directly under the focal point of pain;
4. do not use heat as part of the treatment.

Rear Heel Bruises

Bruises on the back of the heel may be caused by an outside trauma. Being kicked in a soccer or basketball game, or having another player slide into the legs in baseball or soccer can cause a bruise where the Achilles tendon attaches on the back of the heel.

The place where the Achilles tendon attaches has also a vulnerable spot, called the *growth plate*. Pain in this area may be caused by badly fitting shoes, especially if they are too tight, pressing on the back of the heel and bruising it. If the irritation continues, a bone spur may develop. Larger shoes and a doughnut pad can eliminate the pain.

'Pump Bumps'

Retro calcaneal bursitis, or *'pump bumps'*, is a common type of heel bruise. The pain behind the heel is caused by wearing high-heeled shoes, or special sports shoes (specifically for tennis, jogging, and so on), which put extra pressure on the heel. The higher-heel design of many sports shoes often puts additional pressure on the Achilles tendon or the back of the heel and can cause heel pain of this sort. In this condition, the area near the attachment of the Achilles tendon to the heel bone is irritated. This causes some pain.

What to do:

1. use an ice cup in a circular motion to reduce the inflammation;
2. wear shoes with softer heel sections and which do not put pressure on the Achilles tendon. Cut away 'Achilles tabs' at the back of the shoe, or ideally choose shoes without a high tab;
3. use a doughnut pad over the inflamed area;
4. do not do exercises that use the calf muscle (heel raises, jumping, running).

THE PLANTAR

Morton's Neuroma

Morton's Neuroma, or *metatarsalalgia,* occurs on the bottom of the foot where the

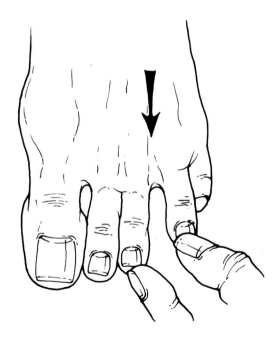

Fig 15. Common location of a neuroma.

toes connect to the foot, at the head of the metatarsals. There is a collection of nerves, or *ganglia,* under the bones at this location, protected by the ball of the foot or the fascia of the plantar surface. The ganglia may be bruised because of trauma or pressure.

If the metatarsal arch (the arch which lies across the foot at the ball of the foot) is not sufficiently high, pressure can be put on the nerves which lie behind the three middle toes. The irritated or swollen nerves can cause pain in the toes or along the sides of the toes, which can be an indication of this condition.

What to do:

1. don't wear narrow or tight shoes;
2. avoid bending the toes backwards during activity (jumping, climbing or descending hills or stairs), and avoid active exercise on hard floors;
3. wear wide stiff shoes to eliminate pinching of the toes and the backward bending of the toes, and use orthotics, arch supports or a pad just behind the ball of the foot;
4. change your exercise from running and jumping to swimming, cycling or rollerblading;
5. R.I.C.E. for half an hour after activity; massage with ice cup;
6. ask a doctor to give a local cortisone injection.

Plantar Fascitis

Plantar fascitis is a common complaint, especially with older athletes. It is an inflammation of the connective tissue under the foot – *plantar* means the bottom of the foot, *fascia* the connective tissue (tendons and ligaments), and *-itis* inflammation – and is said to affect nearly

20 per cent of runners. The soreness is under the foot and in the heel or just forward of the heel. It is usually caused by bruising the tissue on or near the heel. Stepping on a stone is a common cause for runners.

Plantar fascitis may occur in several tissues in the bottom of the foot. The most common area is on or just in front of the heel bone *(calcaneus)*. The ligaments and tendons which attach to the heel are prone to problems from either trauma, over-stretching, or tightening due to not being stretched often enough. Tight calf muscles and tendons *(gastrocnemius and soleus)* are often related, so stretching of the heel is always recommended as part of the cure. Stretching of the rear calf muscles should be done several times a day.

Another contributing factor is often that the foot is pronated or 'flat', with the inside part of the foot closer to the ground. A proper orthotic device or insole, which lifts the long arch of the foot, may help prevent a recurrence.

The pain is particularly noticeable when getting out of bed in the morning, or when arising after being seated for some time. The condition is generally a stress injury in which the tendons under the foot are repeatedly stressed, as in running or in doing heel raises with significant weight on the back. Relative rest is the most important aspect of treatment. A doughnut pad or a rubber heel cup with extra cushioning underneath may also be an aid.

If there is a continuing *plantar fascitis,* it is worth considering your shoe insoles. Most insoles are made for 500 miles of walking or running. The outside and the bottom are made for 800–1,000 miles, so the shoe may look fine, but the major foot-supporting structure may be worn out. Try keeping track of the number of miles shoes have gone, then replace them after 500 miles.

Another way to help get rid of *plantar fascitis* is to use standard treatment: icing after use of the bruised foot, then hot and cold contrasting baths to increase the healing of the tissue in that area. Relative rest is also a good idea, along with a gradual re-introduction of the activity that caused the problem. For example, a runner who commonly runs ten miles a day should cut back to one or two miles daily until the fascitis is cured. Using orthotics and/or rubber heel cups will help to reduce the chance of the problem reoccurring.

What to do:

1. stretch the Achilles tendon by standing a few feet from a wall and allowing your hips to drop towards the wall. Bend the ankle forward and feel the pull at the back of the heel. Do this with the knee bent and straight to stretch the soleus and gastrocnemius, the two muscles of the calf;

2. use a soft rubber heel cup to ease the pain by cushioning the heel bone when the heel hits the floor. The heel cup also reduces the tension of the Achilles tendon and the stretch of the ligaments under the foot;

3. the use of an appropriate orthotic shoe insert may aid recovery;

4. softer, more flexible well-cushioned shoes, rather than stiff shoes, are also generally recommended;

5. NSAIDs, such as aspirin or ibuprofen, may reduce the inflammation and the pain. They mask pain, so care must be taken not to increase training too fast;

6. don't walk or run on your toes, on hard surfaces, walk in bare feet;

7. an injection of corticosteroids may be given if the pain does not ease, and ultrasound or similar techniques of therapy may also speed recovery. In extreme cases, surgery to remove scar tissue and heel spurs may be helpful.

THE TOE

Turf Toe

Turf toe is a bone bruise or ligament sprain at the base of the toe, common to athletes who play on hard surfaces such as Astroturf, concrete or hardwood floors. Real grass allows the athlete to slide while stopping or changing direction, but the hard high-grip surfaces are not so forgiving. The problem may occur in a variety of sports where starting and stopping are frequent, including soccer, basketball, American football, team handball, baseball, softball, or skiing. Lacing shoes properly reduces the risk by reducing the ability of the big toe to slide forward and hit the end of the shoe. This jamming of the foot can bruise both ends of the bones in the big toe and the adjacent toe.

While artificial turf and other hard playing surfaces are generally blamed for the condition, any hyper-extension of the toes, such as when starting to jump, can also cause it, as can a fall, or a trauma to the toe or toe area. In soccer and American football the injury may be caused by a single trauma. In dancers and runners, the injury may be caused by a more chronic and continual bending backward of the toes. Padding, appropriate taping and orthotics may be used to aid in the healing, and orthotics or toe cups may be used to prevent the injury.

The best way to get rid of this condition is to go back to the standard treatment: icing after every workout or game, and contrast-

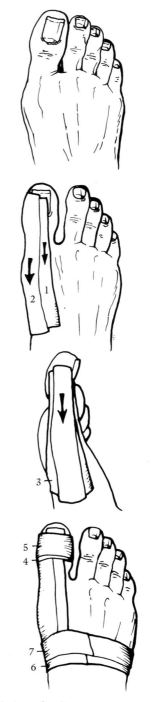

Fig 16. Taping a bunion.

ing baths of cold and hot. To reduce the pain during participation, use some type of adhesive taping to neutralize the movement that causes the most pain. Obviously, the toe can only flex and extend in two directions, but no athlete has the same pain in one direction or the other, so taping to avoid the painful movement would be helpful.

The toe may be taped in different ways. If pain occurs during flexing, tape the foot in a neutral position, so that it cannot flex but can extend. Put several layers of tape above the big toe, extending it from the tip of the toenail to half-way up the top of the foot. Anchor one end by taping around the toe. Anchor the other end by taping around the foot. If the pain occurs when the toe is extending (moving towards the top of the foot) as when standing on tiptoes or landing from a jump, tape below the toe and anchor the tape as above. Make sure shoes are fitted and laced properly, as this may help to eliminate the problem and the pain.

Skier's Toe

Skier's toe is an over-use injury often experienced by cross-country skiers, especially if they have recently changed their skiing technique. It is an inflammation at the base of the big toe.

Hammer Toes

Also called claw toes or curled-up toes, hammer toes are caused by tightened connective tissue (tendons or ligaments) under one or more toes. Some people are born with hammer toes, while others develop them by wearing shoes that are too short. One resultant problem is that the tops of the toes become irritated by any movement of the foot while wearing shoes.

What to do:
1. have the condition corrected by surgery;
2. stretch the toes backwards to stretch the connective tissue under them;
3. wear shoes which are sufficiently long so that the toes can stretch forward, and loose enough so that there is minimal irritation on the top of the shoes;
4. pad the tops of the toes with small doughnut-style pads (available at pharmacies).

Black Toenails

Toenails can appear black when the toes are bruised. Bruising under the toenail is commonly caused by short shoes or shoes that are not laced sufficiently tightly, causing the foot to slide forwards each time you stop. Rugby, soccer, basketball and long-distance running are sports in which this problem is particularly prevalent, but any activity in which the foot slides forwards and hits the end of the shoe can cause it.

Another possibility is that the shoes are too narrow, causing the little toe to have a black toenail due to the toe next to it being squeezed against it. Any growing athlete who uses the same athletic shoes for a long period of time must be aware of potential problems. As feet grow, new shoes are essential!

In-Grown Toenails

This is quite common, but not usually a major problem. The end of the toenail digs under the skin and creates inflammation. This can be prevented by trimming the toenails straight across so that they can't get under the skin. Wider, more comfortable shoes will also reduce the risk of inflammation.

THE TOP OF THE FOOT

The top of the foot can be injured by bruises or tendinitis. There are tendons going across the top of the foot, and a tendinitis may develop from lacing shoes too tightly. One way to determine if the problem is tendinitis is to take off the shoes and try to keep the bottom of the foot on the floor, lifting the toes off the ground as high as possible; or, hold the toes up while someone tries to pull the toes down. If either of these actions cause pain or irritation across the top of the foot, there is probably some tendinitis due to an irritation of the tendon.

All tendons have a sheath around the outside. When the sheath is compressed in the foot with a shoe that is laced too tightly, the sheath becomes irritated and breaks blood vessels, and swelling occurs. Every time the foot is moved or the toes are moved up and down, such as when you walk or run, there will be pain from the tendinitis.

BONE INJURIES

The wrist, the ankle and the foot are similar in that each is made up of a large number of bones. There is, therefore, a great chance of a sprain of the ligaments that hold the bones together, or of a break in one of the bones. The various uses of the foot – providing take-off power in a run or jump, acting as a landing shock absorber in running and jumping, providing the means to change

directions in cutting sports, and as the surface for several types of kick – make the foot and ankle a likely site of sport injury.

Fractures

Fractures of the bones of the feet are common. Falling, being stepped on, or receiving a blow to the foot may cause a bone to break. If there is any doubt, see a doctor and get x-rays. Otherwise, treat the injury as a sprained ankle, with rest, ice, compression, and a brace.

Stress fractures are commonly caused by continued repetitive stresses on the foot bones. Long-distance walking or running are common causes of stress fractures in the foot. The symptoms of stress fractures are pain, particularly increasing pain with increased exercise. A fracture will only heal with rest.

What to do:
1. take the pain seriously. If an activity hurts, especially if it makes you limp, don't do it;
2. see a doctor if the pain does not subside within a few weeks;
3. if necessary, switch to another activity, such as swimming or cycling, if pain persists.

SHOES, ORTHOTICS AND HEEL CUPS

It is evident from the list of possible injuries to the feet that proper shoes are essential for the athlete who walks, runs or jumps. A huge number of styles for every type of athletic event are available, but don't choose a shoe because of its colour, or because it is endorsed by your sporting hero. For example, the high heel tab on the back of many sport shoes may look nice, but it can put extra pressure on the heel and the Achilles tendon.

Shoes should have the proper amount of cushioning for the relevant activity. They begin to lose their efficiency as shock absorbers after 200–500 miles of running, so you may need to buy new shoes before you have worn out the soles of the old ones. Shoes with inflexible soles are a major cause of foot and lower-leg problems.

The proper way to lace a pair of shoes is to put the laces in from the top down, rather than from the bottom up. The only exception is at the top eyelet, where the lace is threaded from the bottom up, because it is easier to tie. If laces go over the top of the eyelet, the laces help hold the shoe snug, and won't loosen. When you put the shoes on, tighten the laces at the bottom eyelets, then tighten them at each succeeding eyelet up to the top eyelet where you tie the shoes. Your foot will be held in a proper position, and should not slide forwards, which might cause black toenails or blisters.

Orthotics are shoe inserts which are generally used to help the heel and arches of the foot. Properly designed, they can prevent and help to heal foot, ankle and lower-leg problems, especially *plantar fascitis,* shin splints, fallen or weak arches. Runners and skiers find them to be helpful in holding the foot in its proper position and in making shoes or boots fit more effectively. Doctors, chiropodists and chiropractors can all fit orthotics, and there are also some that can be bought from sporting goods stores. These are made for the traditional problems in feet, and may not be suitable for every individual.

Heel cups can reduce or prevent some problems. Hard plastic heel cups can make up for poor-fitting heels in your shoes, while soft rubber heel cups can absorb shocks and help to prevent or ease those problems in which continued stresses occur. Heel spurs, *plantar fascitis* and shin splints can be aided by rubber heel cups.

FOOT EXERCISES

1. Curl toes under, then hyperextend them.
2. Abduct and adduct the toes.
3. Pick up marbles or small wads of paper.
4. Curl a towel.
5. Do heel raises (on a board).
6. Perform inversion (inward motion against a hand).
7. Perform eversion (outward motion against a hand).
8. Do Achilles tendon stretch against a wall.

CHAPTER 3
The Ankle and Lower Leg

SPRAINED ANKLE

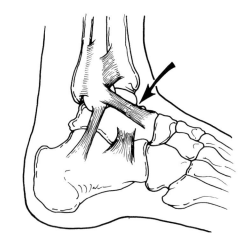

Fig 17. Ankle ligaments: outside view.

The sprained ankle is the most common type of athletic injury. It occurs when the ligaments on the outside of the ankle are severely over-stretched. Ligaments take some time to recover normal length, strength and sensitivity to stretch, so ankle sprains often recur. In fact 75 per cent of people who sprain an ankle will re-sprain it within a year, and this is normally due to inadequate rehabilitation.

While any of the ligaments in the foot or ankle can be sprained, it is most commonly those in the lower outside area of the ankle that are affected. The outside part of the foot moves downwards and the weight of the body stretches the ligaments. People who play basketball, volleyball, or other sports in which they rapidly change direction, are likely to suffer this type of injury. In

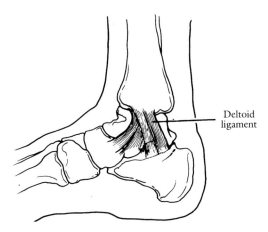

Fig 18. Ankle ligaments: inside view.

Deltoid ligament

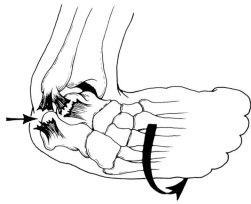

Fig 19. Severe ligament sprain.

soccer or American football, a tackle or block from one side may sprain the ankle on the far side, as the force hits high on the calf, while the cleats of the shoe hold the foot firm on the turf. Uneven playing surfaces can also result in sprained ankles.

Sometimes a 'crack' is heard as the ligament tears. At other times there is only the stretching of the ligaments, followed by immediate pain. Swelling begins almost straightaway. The standard treatment of ice (and, later, heat), compression and elevation should be started immediately. Mild sprains will often be sufficiently healed within a week to allow activities to be resumed. More severe sprains may take six weeks.

Some precautions need to be taken to prevent a re-occurrence of the injury. The ankle may be taped; this has been used in sports such as football and basketball, but an ankle brace may be more effective, as tape often stretches after the first half an hour. The lace-up type of ankle brace, with Velcro straps that add additional support to the ankle, is commonly used, as is the plastic hinged brace. The plastic type is more expensive but does not bind the ankle too tightly, thereby allowing the up and down movement that is essential to running and jumping. In an analysis of several types of ankle braces compared with standard ankle supporting tape (Shapiro *et al,* 'Ankle sprain prophylaxis and analysis of the stabilizing effects of bracing and tape', *AJSM,* Jan 94, page 78), tape ranked only sixth in effectiveness.

'High-top' shoes offer some protection to an ankle prone to sprains, but they reduce the ankle's mobility. Simple tubigrip tubular bandage also gives extra protection, enabling the muscles around the ankle to react quickly to any stretch.

What to do with a sprained ankle:

1. R.I.C.E. several times a day at first, then follow the standard treatment of cold and heat;
2. using thick felt (quarter to half an inch), make a U-shaped pad to go under the ankle bone;
3. use an ankle brace, or adhesive tape, to do the supporting that the ligament would normally do.

Taping

Taping is best done by a chartered physiotherapist or athletic trainer, who would be likely to do the following:

1. put a strip of tape around the lower part of the calf muscle, not making it too tight. This is to anchor the tape;
2. holding the outside of the foot as high as possible, run a strip of athletic training tape downwards from the anchor strip, under the heel, and up to the outside. Repeat this three or four times, slightly overlapping the tape strips. This tape will support the outside of the foot as the torn ligament had been doing;
3. starting at the inside of the ankle, run a strip down under the foot, up, then behind the ankle, then back under the heel, then around the ankle again. This will lock in the strips;
4. an experienced practitioner will always start on the inside of the foot and work to the outside, and will make sure the foot is flexed upwards and outwards.

Exercises

Within a few days, after swelling has stopped, the injured person will be able to swim, cycle, or walk slowly, but should make

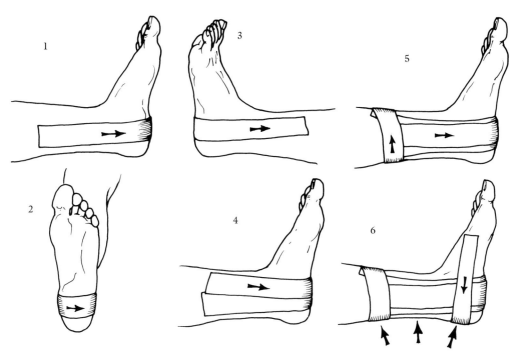

Fig 20. Basic taping of the ankle.

an effort not to limp. Gentle flexing of the ankle can aid in the absorption of the fluids that cause the swelling. Any use of the ankle should be finished with cold and compression. Into the second seventy-two hours of treatment, the number of exercises can be increased, in order to reduce the development of scar tissue. Use some or all of the following:

1. foot circles, pretending there is a ball in front of the big toe, and making the toe go around the outside of the ball, clockwise and anti-clockwise, making circles;
2. pretend the big toe is a pencil and use it to write the alphabet;
3. as the range of motion increases, the towel exercise may be used. Place a towel on the floor under the foot, with the toes at the end of the towel, and pull the towel under the foot, thus strengthening the toes;
4. pick up objects, such as marbles, from the floor with the toes;
5. rise up on the toes, skip with a rope, and hop on both feet;
6. hop on only one foot, then walk and jog, progressing to full mobility.

The ankle should be supported, either with a brace or tape, while the hopping, walking or jogging exercises are done to avoid re-injury. Medical studies show that moving the ankle early after a sprain is generally better than immobilization.

LOWER-LEG INJURIES

Shin Splints

The term shin splints, or medial tibial stress syndrome, describes pain and tenderness in

31

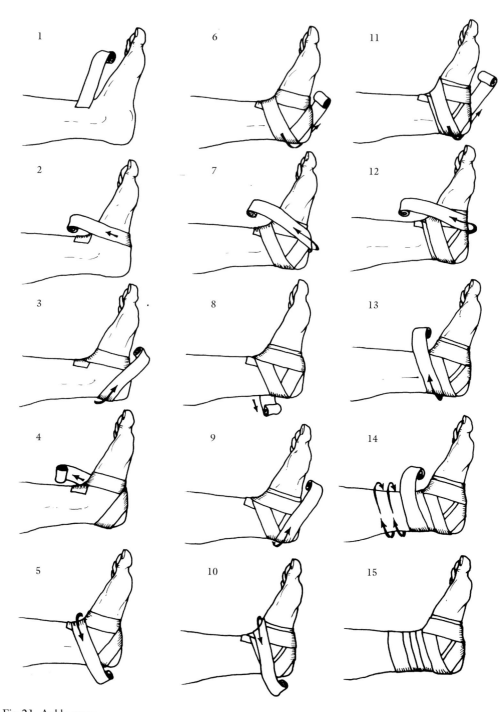

Fig 21. Ankle wrap.

the middle part of the front of the shin bone *(tibia)*. A sharp pain is more likely to be a fracture but pain only on running suggests shin splints. Pre-disposing factors are poor leg or foot alignment, incorrect shoes for the activity, poor running mechanics, running too much (over-training), or running on hard surfaces. Plyometrics, such as box-jumping, can also cause tibial and shin splint problems.

To reduce the chances of developing shin splints, wear shoes that fit properly, and have good shock-absorbing properties. Orthotic inserts to the shoes can also reduce the stress to the leg by holding the foot and arches in the proper position. When the foot is turned inwards, or the arches are not capable of absorbing the shock of continual running, either custom-made orthotics or commer-cially made inserts can be a great aid in reducing foot, ankle and lower-leg prob-lems.

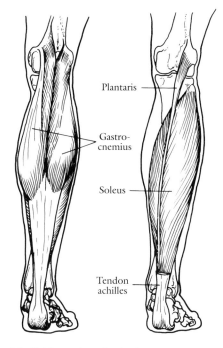

Fig 23. Calf muscles – back view.

The athlete's activity has either caused minute muscle tears, has stretched the con-nective tissue between the muscle fibres, or has overly stretched and damaged the tissues holding the muscle to the shin bone. Determining the cause of the injury enables the sufferer to direct the healing efforts more effectively.

What to do:
1. R.I.C.E., with ice cup massage;
1. strengthen the muscle by moving your foot upwards against the pressure of your hand;
2. wear orthotics or arch supports and/or better-cushioned shoes. Commercial shoe inserts should also help;
3. don't expect shin splints to heal them-selves; they will only get worse if efforts are not made to correct the problem;

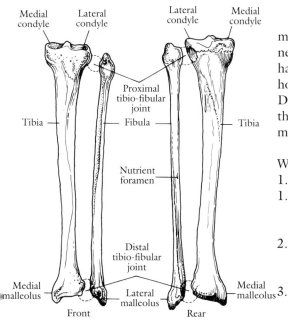

Fig 22. Lower leg.

33

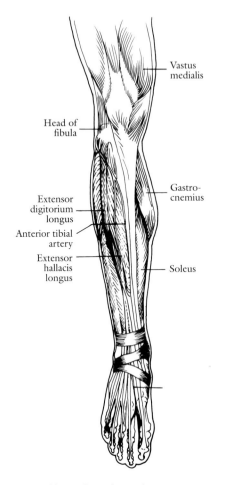

Fig 24. Calf muscles – front view.

Labels on figure:
Vastus medialis
Head of fibula
Extensor digitorium longus
Anterior tibial artery
Extensor hallacis longus
Gastro-cnemius
Soleus

strains are not uncommon, because the calf muscles are used in every running, jumping and dancing activity, as well as in some kicking activities such as soccer and martial arts.

'Tennis leg' is an injury to the tendons of the top of the calf muscle (gastrocnemius), caused by pushing off on the serve, rising on the toes to hit an overhead smash, or pushing off hard to move forwards.

Cramps in the calf are quite common in runners, especially during hot weather, when excessive amounts of fluids have been lost. Swimmers may also experience such cramps when they extend the toes down forcefully or when the water is cold and reduces circulation. In a cramp a large number of the muscle fibres contract and will not relax. Any muscle with insufficient blood can cramp.

What to do:
1. ask someone to help break the cramp for you. Lie on your back, extend the leg up, bend the ankle forward, and let the other person push down on the ball of your foot to break the cramp;
2. sometimes the cramp will re-occur after a short time. Repeat the procedure and massage the muscle to increase the circulation.

4. if the problem is caused by running, run on soft sand or soft grass rather than on a hard track or the road, or rest from running by cross training (cycling or swimming).

The Calf Muscles

Other than shin splints, most lower-leg problems occur in the back of the leg. Paratendonitis, stress fractures and muscle

Fractures

Fracture of the tibia or fibula can occur from repeated stresses or from a single trauma. The single trauma is generally a blow from the side, which may occur when being tackled in soccer or American football or when sliding into a base in baseball.

Stress fractures are more likely to occur in the older athlete, in whom the bone minerals are insufficient (osteoporosis); they are

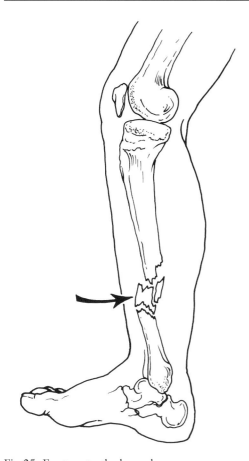

Fig 25. Fracture to the lower leg.

often due to amenorrhoea (*see* Chapter 18), the level of fitness, and the alignment of the legs and feet.

The total number of stress fractures that occur affect the different parts of the body as follows: 34 per cent in the tibia, 24 per cent the fibula, 18 per cent the ankle bones, 14 per cent the thigh bone (femur), 6 per cent the pelvis, and 4 per cent other bones. Female athletes taking part in sports involving landing (jumpers, dancers, gymnasts), or changing direction quickly and frequently (basketball, soccer, handball) are more likely to develop stress fractures of the fibula. Female long-distance runners are more likely to develop stress fractures of the tibia. The 'female athlete triad' is considered to be a primary factor in fractures in women (see Chapter 18).

Running on a slanted surfaces, for example, on the side of the road where the slope is usually away from the road, or on a banked track, is more likely to cause problems in the 'uphill' leg. For this reason, it is best to balance the leg stress by running out and back on the same side of the street, or running in both directions on the embanked track. Running on a soft surface, such as grass or sand, significantly reduces the forces that the tibia and the surrounding muscles and tendons must absorb.

The Achilles Tendon

Achilles tendinitis or rupture is quite common. The muscles in the back of the calf are extremely strong and are used in nearly every movement – walking, running, jumping, dancing or skiing. These muscles control the tension on the Achilles tendon (heel cord). With every step or jump, tension is put on the heel cord and problems can result. A series of minor injuries can develop into a chronic *paratendonitis*. The same type of force that can injure the tendon can also injure the muscle fibres and strain or tear them.

What to do:

1. R.I.C.E., followed by the standard treatment of heat and cold;
2. use heel pads or an elevated heel cup to reduce the stretch on the tendon;
3. shift to an exercise programme that does not stretch the Achilles tendon. Swimming is preferred, but weight training would also be a possibility, as would cycling, if the ankle is not allowed to extend.

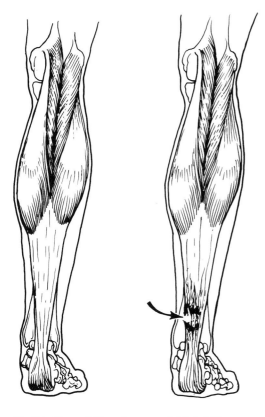

Fig 26. Normal (l) and ruptured (r) Achilles tendon.

During vigorous activity the Achilles tendon may completely tear. This feels like a sudden sharp blow to the calf followed by severe pain. Urgent surgical treatment is needed.

Exercises for the Lower Leg
1. To strengthen the outside of the ankle, sit in a chair with one leg crossed over the other. With your hand, put pressure on the outside of the foot and move the foot outwards (eversion).
2. Now put your hand against the top part of your toes and lift your foot upwards (inversion).
3. Toe raises (going up on the toes) will help to strengthen the muscles in the back of the ankle. It is better to do these one leg at a time, to double the bodyweight that your calf muscle must lift.

CHAPTER 4
The Knee

The knee is a much-used body part in most sports, and the most commonly injured joint, damaged either by direct blows or twists, which stretch ligaments, or by chronic actions, which can bruise or otherwise injure the internal surfaces of the joint. Direct blows to the knee, for example, are most likely to stretch ligaments and may also injure the *menisci*, the semi-circular cartilage-like cushions that ease the sliding of the thigh bone (femur) on the leg bone (tibia).

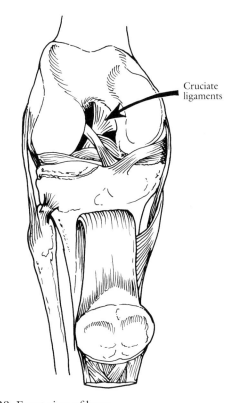

Fig 28. Front view of knee.

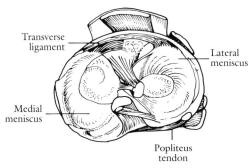

Fig 27. Top view of knee.

THE MENISCUS (CARTILAGE)

Cartilage *(meniscus)* injuries are most likely to occur when the leg is planted firmly on the ground and the knee twisted hard. The torn meniscus may cause locking and swelling of the knee joint in certain situations, and locking is generally a sign of a cartilage injury. Generally, surgical repair is required (about 30 per cent of such injuries are self-healing). Whether or not surgery is used, the muscles that stabilize the knee must be strengthened by knee flexion, extension exercises and calf extensions. Bicycle riding is also very helpful.

THE KNEE LIGAMENTS

The *cruciate* (meaning 'in the shape of a cross') *ligaments* are inside the knee joint and protect the knee against excessive forward-backward movement. The ability to control a knee with a torn anterior cruciate ligament depends on leg muscle strength and co-ordination, and the stresses of the sport.

Severe strain on the knee can damage the cruciate ligaments and the menisci and can also stretch the ligaments on the sides of the knee, which prevent excessive side-to-side motion. Generally, a blow from the outside would push the knee inwards and stretch or tear the inside *(medial collateral)* ligament. Similarly, a bend of the knee outwards, perhaps caused by a blow from the inside, would stretch the outside *(lateral collateral)* ligament.

It is not only a blow to the knee that can cause injury. Changing direction quickly, as in basketball or soccer, can place enough force on the knee to stretch or tear the ligaments. Sixteen per cent of soccer injuries to men and 19 per cent to women are to the cruciate ligament. It is also common in basketball but, in this sport, women suffer four times as many anterior cruciate sprains as men.

Thirty per cent of skiing injuries are to the knee, which, unlike the ankle, is not protected by the boot. The anterior cruciate and the medial collateral ligaments are the most at risk for skiers, and the forward twisting fall is the most dangerous type of fall. Skiers must therefore make sure that they have bindings that effectively release sideways, and are properly adjusted for the skier's weight and skiing ability. (See Hull, M.L., 'Analysis of Skiing Accidents', *AJSM*, Feb. 1997, p. 35.)

If the injured sportsperson takes part in sports where quick changes of movement are required, such as soccer, rugby, American football, basketball, or team handball, surgery is often advised for cruciate ligament injuries. In other sports, such as swimming or golf, knee control may be adequate after the injury.

While sudden acute trauma to the leg or knee is the most common cause of injury, breast-stroke swimmers often develop 'breast-stroker's knee'. The chronic inward frog kick can put too much continued strain on the ligaments on the inside of the knee.

What to do for any knee ligament or cartilage injury:
1. use the standard treatment (R.I.C.E.);
2. splint if necessary for support;
3. do not twist the leg, do a deep squat, or completely straighten the leg, because this can put unnecessary pressure on the knee ligaments;
4. do not do activities which increase the pain in the knee (such as running or strength training);
5. use crutches or a cane if necessary.

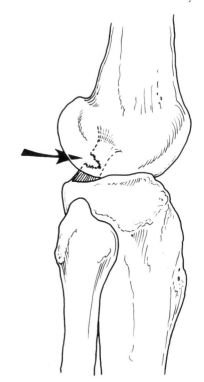

Fig 29. Cruciate ligament tear.

THE KNEE CAP

The knee cap *(patella)* is a bone inside the tendon that attaches the quadriceps muscle in the front of the thigh to the front top of the lower leg bone (tibia). The patella rides in grooves in the knee. A dislocated or sub-luxed patella, when the patella slips sideways out of its channels, is a not uncommon problem, especially in those who have small-er bone ridges or weak quadriceps, or have already suffered injury. The most likely caus-es of the patella slipping to the side are a direct blow to the front or the inside of the knee cap, or a twisting of the thigh when the lower leg is firmly anchored on the ground.

What to do:
1. have the knee cap re-set by a doctor if it is out of place;
2. use the standard treatment;
3. wear a special knee-cap brace to prevent a re-occurrence;
4. strengthen the thigh muscles (quadri-ceps).

PATELLIOFEMORAL PAIN SYNDROME

Less serious knee pain can affect every aspect of the knee. Below are some of the problems commonly experienced.

Anterior Knee Pain

Pain under the knee cap (patella) is medical-ly termed 'anterior knee pain' (pain in the front of the knee). It is the most common over-use injury of the knee. There are many pre-disposing factors, including the mis-alignment of the knee cap caused by a lack of flexibility, muscular weakness in the

quadriceps, bone deformity, or a roughening of the smooth cartilage lining of the patella which doesn't allow it to ride smoothly in its most desired track.

'Housemaid's Knee'

Pain at the front of the knee, commonly referred to as 'housemaid's knee', with swelling and pain on top of the knee cap, is caused by repetitive trauma inflicted by activities such as kneeling.

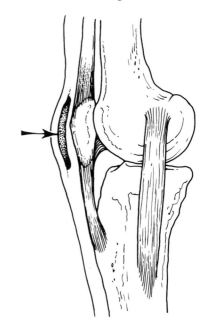

Fig 30. Side view of 'housemaid's knee'.

'Jumper's Knee'

Patellar tendonitis ('jumper's knee') is com-mon at all ages among runners and jumpers. The continued flexion and extension of the knee joint during running can cause minute damage to the tendon. In more severe cases the tendon can tear in the area of the patella,

39

or closer to the tendon's attachment below the knee.

Osgood-Schlatter's Disease

This complaint is often found in young people, usually aged from 12 to 15, who have been active in running and jumping. The tissue that will become bone as the child matures is still soft. The continued running and jumping puts great strain on the patellar tendon at its insertion below the knee. The softer tissue of the tibia may be pulled outwards and a bump on the tibia develops. It is usually quite painful and several months of reduced activity are required, often until the bone is fully mature.

Pain at the Side of the Knee Cap

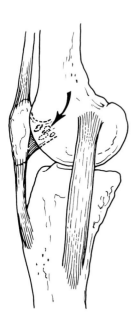

Pain, and possibly snapping, at the side of the knee cap may be caused by a thickened *plica*. This is a tissue that is attached to the lower front of the femur and to the patellar area. As it stiffens it may cause pain, and perhaps snapping, when the knee bends. Bending the knee, as when doing squats, getting up from a

Fig 31. Bone chips in knee.

chair, or climbing stairs may bring on the pain or snapping.

Iliotibial Band Syndrome

Pain and snapping at the outside of the knee ('iliotibial band syndrome') is caused by the end of the iliotibial band of connective tissue being over-used and irritated. The snapping occurs when the end of the band moves over a raised portion of the tibia. Poor running technique or too much running may contribute to this problem.

Pain at the Back of the Knee

Pain in this area of the knee may be due to inflamed hamstring tendons or bursa (the fluid-filled sac).

Pain Inside the Knee

This kind of pain is due to a number of causes, including cartilage or bone damage. *Osteochondritis dissecans* is caused by one or more pieces of bone separating from the original site. Pieces frequently separate themselves from the thigh bone, and these small bone chips (sometimes called 'joint mice') can damage the inside of the knee and cause pain and even a locking of the knee. The condition often requires surgery.

What to do for knee pain:
1. use the standard treatment;
2. reduce the bending of the knees (avoid doing squats, climbing stairs, etc);
3. wear a patellar brace if the patella is involved in the movements that are causing the pain;

4. where incorrect running or running on hard surfaces is the cause of the problem use orthotics and/or shoes with more cushioning.

KNEE BRACES

A knee brace may help in preventing a first injury or re-injury to the knee. However, the research is not conclusive, and a simple tubular elastic bandage that enhances proprioception – improving the speed of reaction to unpredicted movements – is probably as effective. It will also help reduce swelling. While a braced knee can clearly withstand more sideways pressure in a static position than an unbraced knee, in sports the knee is almost never in a static position. Large-scale studies in the USA on football players have sometimes shown braces to have a preventive effect.

On the other hand, there are studies that have shown the occurrence of more injuries when the knee is braced. It has been hypothesized that this is due to muscle fatigue, caused by the straps that hold the brace in position cutting circulation, so that fatigue occurs earlier. It may also be because the weight of the brace tires the braced leg sooner – a 5 per cent increase in energy use due to the brace has been recorded. The initial protection potential of the brace is reduced as fatigue sets in during a practice or competition.

TREATMENT FOR A KNEE JOINT INJURY

The only movement of the knee joint is flexion-extension. At the beginning, when movement is limited, put the knee in ice and move it as far as possible. Then work on the muscles that extend (straighten) and the muscles that flex (bend), by doing some skipping, walking, jogging, and working on a weight machine doing leg extensions and leg curls.

EXERCISES

Correct squats (knee bends), straight-leg raises, side-leg raises (abduction and adduction), standing hip flexion, lying hip extension, sitting knee extension, standing knee flexion, toe raises, quadriceps setting.

CHAPTER 5
The Hip, Pelvis and Thigh

THE HIP

The Tendons

Injuries to the tendons of the hips and their insertions into the hip bones are common in adolescent athletes. A violent contraction of the muscles at the same time that they are being stretched (an eccentric contraction as part of the 'stretch-shortening cycle') can injure either the tendon or the bone. Sports in which the legs are forced to move quickly,

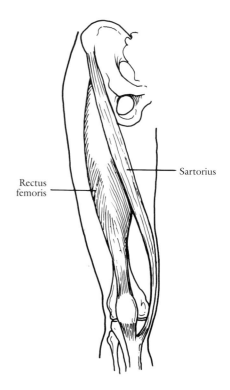

Fig 33. Exterior muscles at front of thigh (flex hips)

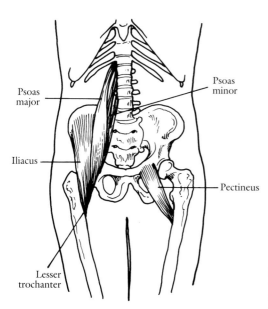

Fig 32. Deep hip flexing muscles.

such as sprinting or slalom skiing, are the most likely culprits. Surgery may or may not be required, but four to six weeks of rest is generally mandatory. Treatment will require NSAIDs (non-steroidal anti-inflammatory drugs, such as aspirin or ibuprofen), ice, and resting in a position which does not strain the injured area.

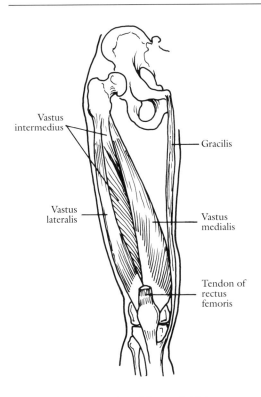

Vastus intermedius

Gracilis

Vastus lateralis

Vastus medialis

Tendon of rectus femoris

Fig 34. Interior muscles of front of thigh (extend knee).

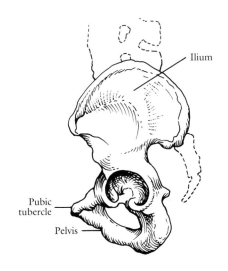

Ilium

Pubic tubercle

Pelvis

Fig 35. Hip bone: side view.

Fractures

Great force is needed to break a normal hip bones, as they are very strong. Hip fractures can be acute, caused by a single blow, or they can be chronic, the result of continued stresses. They are particularly likely to occur in long-distance women runners who are not having periods. The most likely sports for hip fractures are horseback riding, downhill skiing, and cycling; in all of these, bad falls are likely to happen. Surgery is normally needed for a hip fracture.

Strains

Strains to the adductor muscles (the muscles under the hips that bring the thighs closer to the body) are relatively common in skiers (both downhill and cross country), and hockey players. They can also occur when quick inward movements of the legs are made: for example, kicking a soccer ball, moving sideways in American football, performing a lateral split jump in figure skating, gymnastics, and many forms of dance. As with other muscular injuries, ice, heat, rest, and ultrasound can be used. Gradual strengthening and stretching must also be started after the pain has been reduced.

Bursitis

Bursitis in the trochanteric area (joint of the thigh bone and the hip) is often found in long-distance runners, especially women. Poor running technique, especially swaying side to side or having the feet cross the midline of the body, is often a cause. Tightened thigh muscles, both hamstrings and quadriceps, as well as tightened gluteal muscles, are also often linked to the problem. The tradi-

43

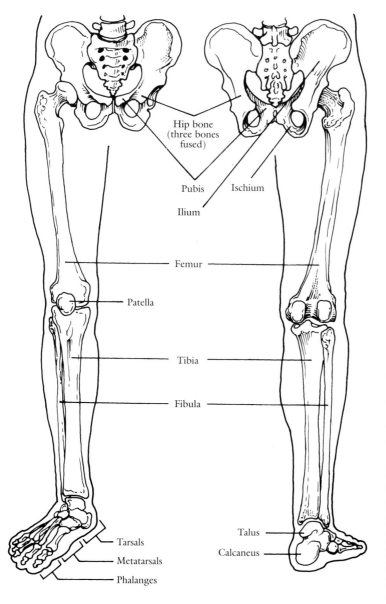

Fig 36. Hip and leg front (l) and rear (r) views.

tion is needed. The athlete should substitute swimming or cycling for running for a time. Once the bursitis is healed, the athlete should seek to increase flexibility and strength.

Bursitis in the buttocks can be caused by a fall on the buttocks or by chronic pressure in the area. Sometimes the pain is not really bursitis and comes from the lower back. If the problem persists, the sufferer should see a doctor.

Snapping Hip Condition

This condition may have a number of causes, but a tight *iliopsoas* muscle is perhaps the most common. Another cause is the *tensor fascia lata* moving over the hip joint as the thigh is moved forwards and back. There may also be soft-tissue injury that allows a muscle to move from its normal place. Runners, gymnasts, hurdlers and dancers are the most commonly afflicted. Treatment requires rest and physical therapy modalities.

tional treatment of ice and heat should help, as will physiotherapy, and occasionally injec-

THE PELVIS

The Pubic Region

Injuries to this region, the lower front of the hip bone and torso, can be caused by a direct blow, but can also develop with a continued overload to the area. Endurance athletes – cross-country skiers, long-distance runners – as well as team-sport players in soccer, team handball, and ice hockey, are often afflicted by such problems. The pain may be due to an inflamed tendon, tendon attachment to bone, or a stress fracture *(osteitis pubis)*. This is often thought to be a chronic adductor strain, but is, in fact, more serious.

The Front of the Hip Joint

Pain at the front of the hip joint can be caused by a stress fracture, tendinitis *(iliopsoas tendinitis)*, or an avulsive fracture. These problems are generally related to over-training, with the body enduring too much of an exercise load. This can occur at the beginning of a training programme, or after a number of months at a high level of exercise.

What to do for pelvis injuries:
1. use the standard treatment;
2. stop any exercise which causes pain;

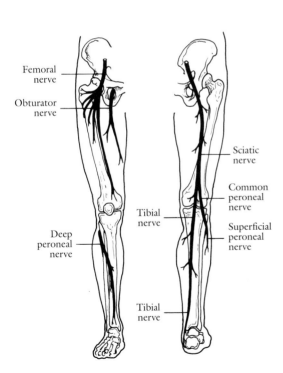

Fig 37. Major nerves of the leg.

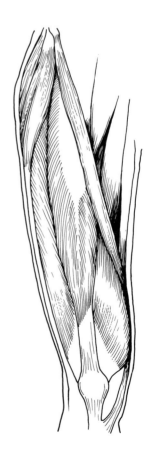

Fig 38. Quadriceps.

3. if tight clothes cause additional pain, wear loose clothes;
4. do hip stretches, and exercises to build up hip strength.

THE THIGH

Muscle Pulls

Pulls (also called strains or tears) are common in the hamstrings (muscles at the back of the thigh), and occur classically in sprinters and jumpers. The pain is generally in the belly of the muscle. The damage is most likely to occur when the athlete is running fast and quickly has to change the direction of the thigh, from being pulled forwards by the quadriceps to being pulled backwards by the hamstrings. The more speed the athlete has generated, the more quickly this action must occur. The small muscle fibres may not be able to bear the transition and may become strained. Often, the sufferer has not warmed up properly, or is fatigued and therefore losing co-ordination, and the hamstrings may be weak relative to the quadriceps. Injuries are nearly always to the weaker hamstring. (Orchard, J. *et al*, 'Pre-season hamstring muscle weakness associated with hamstring muscle injury', 15.118 Feb 97, p. 81).

While muscle pulls in the hamstrings are likely to be high in the muscle, pulls in the quadriceps (front of the thigh) are likely to be lower in the muscle and may occur near, or in, the patellar tendon.

What to do:
1. use the standard treatment;
2. stretch the muscles slowly if there is no pain; do not over-stretch. Stretching will reduce the formation of scar tissue and prevent shortening of the muscle body. This may begin after 3 to 4 days;
3. do strengthening and stretching exercises to help the recovery;
4. return to the sport after this type of injury may take four weeks or longer.

Proprioceptive Neuro-muscular Facilitation (PNF) is an effective (but potentially dangerous) hamstring stretching technique done with a partner. One athlete lies on the ground, with the partner standing. The partner on the ground lifts one leg up as far as possible and then tries to push it back down

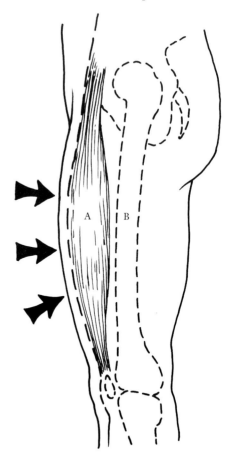

Fig 39. Common sites of quadricep pulls.

to the ground, against the standing partner, for ten seconds. The leg is then more relaxed and can be passively stretched further by the standing partner.

Bruises

Bruises of the thigh muscles are common, especially in contact sports, and the quadriceps are particularly vulnerable. These bruises ('Charlie horses') can be on the surface or deep. The deeper bruises are accompanied by a rupture of the blood vessels in the area of the bruise. This causes a *haematoma* (a collection of blood, usually clotted) which can be very serious, especially if the muscle is exercised further. Its most serious consequence can be the formation of bone bits in the muscle. This is called *myositis ossificans*.

What to do:
1. use the standard treatment and elevate the joint, with the knee bent, to reduce blood pooling in the bruised area;
2. stop all lower-body exercise; such exercise can increase the blood pooling and the possibility of *myositis ossificans;*
3. use firm compression to reduce swelling.

Fractures

A fracture of the thigh bone (femur) usually happens with a single blow, but stress fractures are also possible in sports such as long-distance running and triathlon (especially in

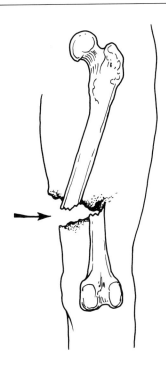

Fig 40. Compound fracture of the femur.

women with few or no menstrual periods). The stress fracture will usually feel like a generalized pain in the thigh and probably not like the sharp pain associated with a complete fracture.

EXERCISES FOR THE HIP, PELVIS AND THIGH

Quad and hamstring stretches (knee bend and hip bend), sitting toe touch, sitting straddle with stretch, abductor stretch, hip strengthening.

CHAPTER 6
The Abdomen

Abdominal injuries account for about 10 per cent of all sports-related injuries.

INJURY FROM A BLOW

An abdominal injury can be caused by either a blunt or a penetrating force. In sport, the great majority of such injuries are caused by blunt forces such as being hit by, or falling on, a ball, or being kicked. Falls from a horse or bicycle, or while rock climbing or auto racing, can also cause injuries to the abdominal viscera.

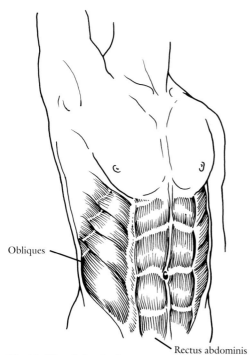

Obliques

Rectus abdominis

Fig 41. The abdominal area.

The injuries can be to the abdominal wall, the muscles and other tissues, or to internal organs such as the liver, spleen or kidneys. The area of injury should be located before a victim is moved, since internal injuries might be accompanied by internal bleeding that could be quite serious. Any bruise to the muscles or the organs can cause bleeding and possibly a *haematoma* (blood pooling or clotting).

STRAINS

Muscle strains to the abdominal wall can occur when the abdominal muscles contract forcefully in jumping or in a twisting movement. Muscular spasms or cramping may occur. The area injured is easily identifiable, as the sharp pain is usually localized.

'STITCH'

A 'stitch' in the side often occurs early in an exercise activity. The precise cause is not known, but the problem may be related to a cramp in the diaphragm due to poor conditioning or poor circulation; it is sometimes assumed to be due to eating shortly before the exercise; it may also be related to weak abdominal muscles. While the pain may be intense, it rapidly subsides with rest. To ease the pain, the torso should be bent away from the side with the pain, and the arm on the side of the pain extended over the head. This should stretch the cramped muscle.

'WINDING'

Being 'winded' is caused by a short-term injury to the abdomen that may affect the diaphragm, the major breathing muscle. If no other injury is evident, one measure to take is to stand over the athlete and slowly pick up the hips by lifting on the belt or waistband. This allows the abdominal organs to push against the diaphragm and helps to expel the air in the lungs. Then the hips should be allowed to return to the floor. The air cavity thereby expands and air is taken into the lungs. A few repetitions will usually suffice to get the athlete breathing normally again.

BRUISES

Bruises to the abdominal wall should be treated in the same way as any other bruises. Be aware of the possibility of bruises or other damage to the organs that lie under the abdominal muscles.

What to do:
1. use the standard treatment;
2. avoid stretching unless it is a cramp;
3. avoid any movement that is painful.

HERNIA

Abdominal hernias can be caused by congenital or acquired weakness. They are more common in men than in women. Hernias in the groin area make up about 75 per cent of all abdominal hernias and are twenty-five times more common in men than in women. If there is a weak area in the abdominal wall or in the pubic area, a small part of the intes-

tine can be pushed through the weakened area. In males, the area in the lower hips where the testicles descend early in life is weakened. This results in a greater frequency of hernias for boys and men.

Lifting a heavy weight, particularly when holding the breath, can often cause the intestine to move through a weakened area in the groin. Holding the breath increases the pressure in the chest, and this is transferred downwards so that there is increased pressure in the abdomen. This is the reason why exhaling while lifting is recommended. The problem is that it is possible to lift more if the breath is held, as the torso is better stabilized; however, in strength training (other than in Olympic lifting), exhalation is recommended. Surgery is almost universally a cure for hernia, and recovery takes three to six weeks on average.

FOOTBALLER'S GROIN

Footballer's groin lasts for weeks or months, often radiating to the lower abdomen or testes, and is due to a hernia-like weakness in the stomach muscles caused by repetitive strain. Suspect this condition (or a stress fracture) if a groin strain does not improve after several months. Surgery is normally needed.

THE SPLEEN

Spleen injuries make up about 50 per cent of all internal abdominal injuries. There can be significant internal bleeding, and pain in the upper left part of the abdomen. A rapid heart rate and low blood pressure can also signal internal bleeding.

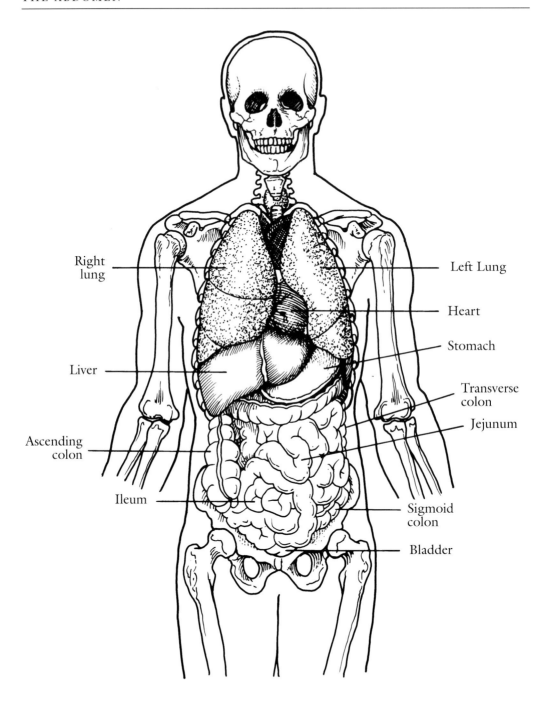

Right lung

Left Lung

Heart

Stomach

Liver

Transverse colon

Jejunum

Ascending colon

Ileum

Sigmoid colon

Bladder

Fig 42. Internal organs.

THE LIVER

Liver injuries account for about 25 per cent of internal abdominal injuries. A direct blow to the right upper part of the abdomen is the most likely cause. It can cause a bruise or a more severe injury that can burst the liver. Muscle spasms and nausea, as well as shock, are possible symptoms of liver injury. Most liver injuries can be treated with bed rest, but some may be severe, requiring blood transfusions or an operation, so a doctor should always be consulted.

THE KIDNEYS

The kidneys can be easily injured by a blow to the lower back area. Boxing and kick boxing, as well as other martial arts and collision games such as football, can damage the kidneys.

THE BLADDER

Injuries to the urinary bladder are rare but do occur. There is a greater chance of their occurrence if the bladder is full. Minor bruises have been found in joggers and marathon runners because of the continued jarring of the bladder by the abdominal organs as each step is taken. A few days of inactivity are generally enough to allow the bruise to heal.

THE STOMACH AND INTESTINES

Injuries to the stomach and intestines are not common and are generally mild. However, if a deep penetrating blow to the abdomen forces the intestines against the spinal column, a rip can occur and a very serious injury can result.

THE GENITALS

The risk of injury to the genitals, particularly the testicles, can be greatly reduced by the use of a protective cup or 'box'. However, a blow can still result in injury and pain. Immediate relief can often be had by lifting and lowering the hips, using the same measure taken when a player is 'winded'. Injuries to the female genitals are more likely to be either bruises or cuts.

What to do with abdominal injuries
1. apply ice to the abdominal area to reduce blood flow to the potentially injured organ;
2. contact a doctor or hospital immediately;
3. stop strength training.

EXERCISES FOR THE ABDOMEN

Curl-ups, crunches, twisting sit-ups. (See Chapter 22).

CHAPTER 7
The Chest and Shoulder

THE CHEST

The Ribs

Rib injuries, including fractures and bruises, are the most common type of chest injury. The ribs should be x-rayed to determine the extent of any injury. If the fracture is not displaced (the bone separated), simply resting for six weeks can generally heal the bone. However, taping or other bracing may be required.

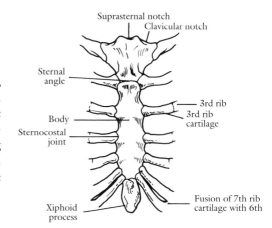

Fig 44. Front view of sterness.

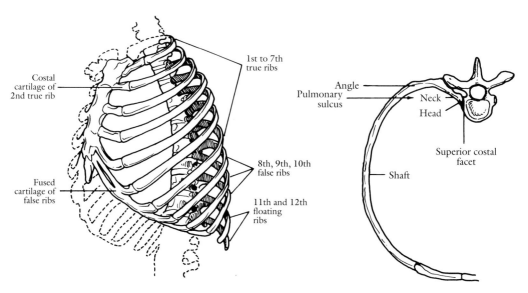

Fig 43. Side view of rib cage.

Fig 45. Top view of rib cage.

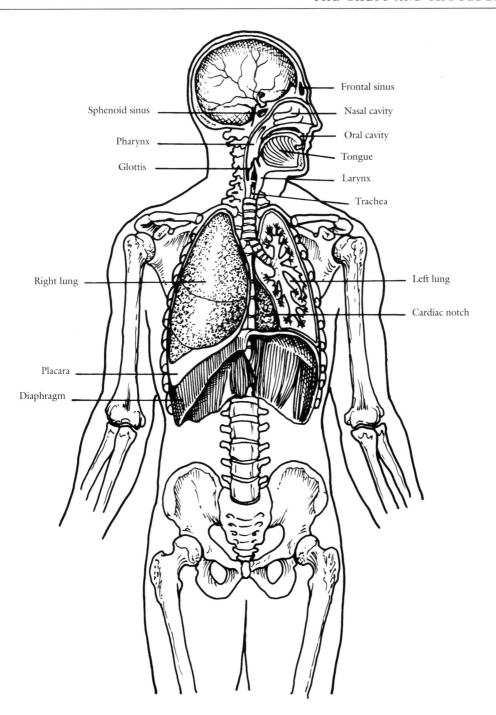

Fig 46. The respiratory system.

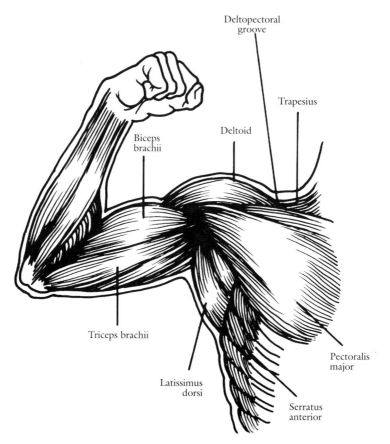

Fig 47. Muscles of the chest and shoulder.

What to do:
1. use the standard treatment;
2. avoid painful activity;
3. consider taping or bracing;
4. breathe as deeply as possible.

Middle Chest

Middle chest pain may appear to come from the ribs or the heart. Often, it is merely from the connective tissues that hold the ribs to the breast bone *(sternum);* this is not seri-ous. The pain may be referred from the back where the ribs join the spine.

Exercises for the Chest

Shoulder stretching in all directions, rotator cuff, forward raise, sideways raise (standing flys), biceps, triceps, push-ups.

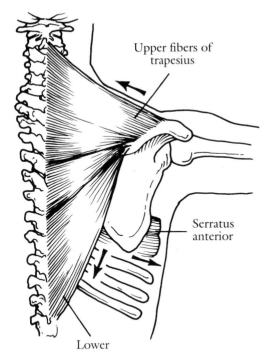

Fig 48. Muscles of the upper back.

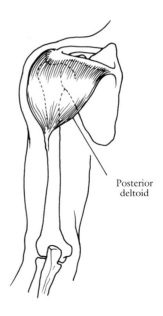

Fig 50

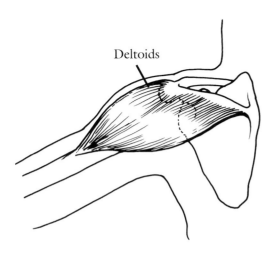

Fig 49. Deltoid abducting humerus.

THE SHOULDER

The shoulder is the most complex of the joints commonly used in sports, giving the body the capacity to move the arm in every direction and to rotate it.

Fracture of the Collar Bone

The collar bone, or *clavicle*, can be fractured as a result of direct trauma, as in American football, when players sometimes fall using a straight arm to break the fall. It can also be the result of accumulated stresses, which build up in weight lifting and shooting sports, for example.

Since the break is usually in the middle of the bone, pushing gently on one end or the other may elicit pain at the fractured area. This test may be used to give an idea as to the type and severity of the injury, but x-rays are always a good idea. The severity of the break will determine whether surgery is

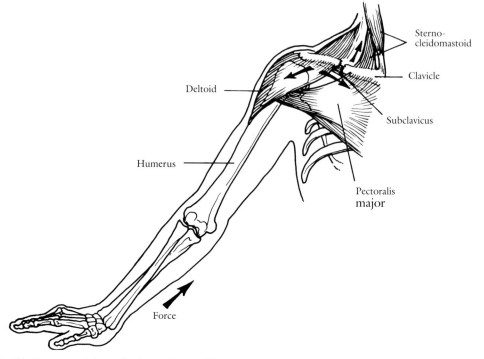

Fig 51. Fracture of the collar bone due to fall.

necessary. Return to sport can generally be made within eight to twelve weeks.

Nerves

Nerve injuries to the upper arm are often called 'burners' or 'stingers'. They are commonly found in football, rugby and ice hockey participants. They may occur because of a blow to, or stretching of, the nerves. A sling may be helpful in reducing the pain. The sportsperson can return to play as soon as the pain has subsided.

Separation or Dislocation

Shoulder separations or dislocations can occur in any direction, but are most com-

monly forwards (anteriorly). Once a dislocation has occurred, it is highly likely to happen again; the ligaments that hold the humerus in the joint formed by the scapula and the clavicle are severely stretched. For that reason, surgery is often needed and a strengthening exercise programme is always essential after an initial period of rest.

Acromioclavicular dislocation is a dislocation of the clavicle where it joins the shoulder, and is normally caused by a fall onto the point of the shoulder. There is no permanent effect on function but there may be a permanent 'step' deformity.

Rotator Cuff

The rotator cuff muscles, which twist the upper arm and stabilze the shoulder joint,

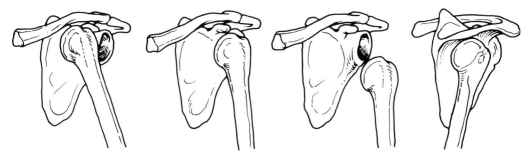

Fig 52. Shoulder dislocations.

are relatively easily injured as the result of muscle tears from stretching or contracting. A hard throwing action, the stopping of a rotation, as when a golfer hits the ground with the club head, or a violent pulling backwards of the upper arm (which might occur in a fall) are all possible causes of a rotator cuff injury. Pain from the injury may be localized or may be felt as far away as the wrist.

When throwing a ball hard, the rotation of the humerus can be more than 7,000 degrees per second – the equivalent to twenty complete 360-degree rotations in a second. Obviously, this puts an enormous strain on these small muscles. All overhead sports ath-

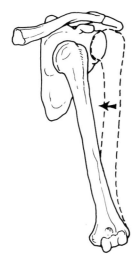

Fig 53. Upper arm completely dislocated.

letes can have rotator cuff problems, but tennis, volleyball, badminton, cricket and baseball players are most likely to suffer. The incidence increases after the age of 35 years.

What to do:
1. apply ice;
2. rest, and then do rotator cuff strengthening exercises;
3. surgery or cortico-steroid injections are sometimes indicated;
4. recovery may take a year or longer.

Chronic Over-Use Syndrome

Complaints relating to this syndrome, such as 'swimmer's shoulder', result from the continued use of the shoulder muscles, and particularly the rotator cuff and the biceps.

Half of all young competitive swimmers, 65 per cent of older swimmers and 70 per cent of elite swimmers have had some problems with the shoulder. It may be a severe inflammation of the tendons *(tendinitis)* or a more chronic variety of the problem (tendinosis). It may also be caused by a swelling of the rotator cuff muscles which limits the movement of the shoulder. It can even be damage to the ends of the upper arm bone, or bone chips in the joint.

While chronic over-use syndrome is quite common among swimmers, it also afflicts

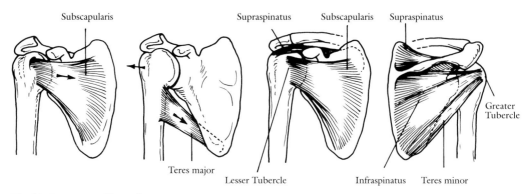

Fig 54. Rotator cuff muscles.

some athletes who continually throw (base-ball pitchers, javelin throwers, bowlers), or hit (badminton or tennis players).

Because there may be several causes it is wise to see a doctor who may order an x-ray.

Stiffness

A stiff shoulder can occur because of an inflammation of the lubricating sac in the shoulder (bursitis), or can be a result of over-use.

What to do with shoulder injuries:
1. ice;
2. rest;
3. then, perform slow movements, build-ing up to full shoulder exercises.

Exercises for the Shoulder

Rotator cuff, all flys (standing, bent, supine), lat pull-downs.

CHAPTER 8
The Neck and the Back

THE NECK

Neck injuries include very serious spinal fractures and spinal dislocations, but also muscle strains and sprains of the ligaments. The muscles to the rear of the spinal column are stronger than those in the front, but a neck bending forwards will be stopped when the chin hits the chest. Serious forward-moving injuries are, therefore, not common. On the other hand, when the neck is extended backwards, it could hyperextend back until the head hits the upper back.

Backward extension of the neck is a far worse problem than forward extension. It can rupture the back part of the disc that separates the vertebral bones, and this can be quite serious.

A whiplash injury in a car or sports accident can stretch the ligaments in the front of the vertebrae, as well as rupturing a disc or two.

An additional note: the increasing number of participants in sports for the disabled, such as the Special Olympics, may need to take special precautions. For example, as many as 40 per cent of Down's Syndrome people may have abnormalities in the cervical area. They need a pre-

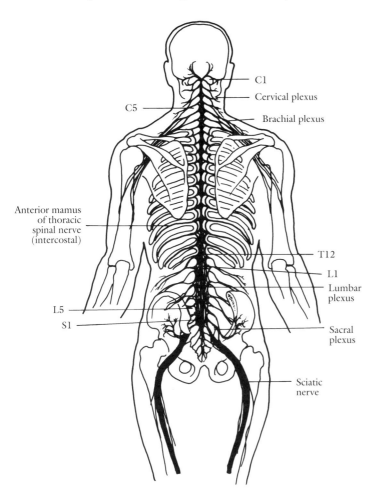

Fig 55. Nerves and the spinal column.

C1
Cervical plexus
C5
Brachial plexus
Anterior mamus of thoracic spinal nerve (intercostal)
T12
L1
Lumbar plexus
L5
S1
Sacral plexus
Sciatic nerve

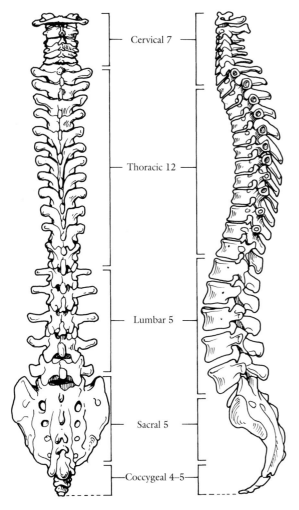

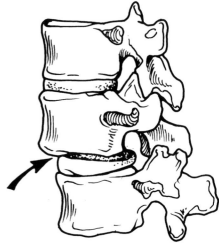

Fig 58. Dislocated vertebra.

ventive examination, as head or neck injuries might occur in activities such as heading the ball in soccer, diving, or falling.

SERIOUS NECK INJURIES

Compression of the Vertebrae

Compression of the vertebrae and discs can be caused by a fall or a blow in which the force comes to the top of the head, especially when the head is bent forward 20 to 30 degrees. Such a blow, caused by a fall from a horse or a cycle, or by poor blocking technique in American football, can shatter a vertebra and possibly a disc, even sending fragments into the spinal cord.

This compression fracture is the most common reason for spinal cord injury and its resulting

Fig 56. Spinal column, rear and side views.

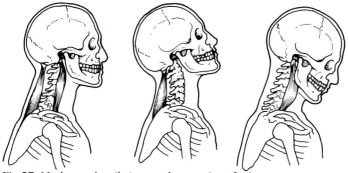

Fig 57. Neck muscles: (l-r) normal, extension, flexion.

paralysis. It is not only found in American football and riding, but also in diving, rugby, gymnastic falls (including tumbling and trampoline falls), and hockey head injuries.

When the injury is to the side of the head, there can be a compression of the vertebrae on the opposite side of the neck. Pain, burning, or tingling may be experienced along the arm, and possibly in the hand. This 'burner' may last several seconds.

Possible Paralysis

One of the greatest concerns with neck injuries is that a bone chip may be loosened and penetrate the spinal cord, causing paralysis, and particularly quadriplegia. The large bone protrusions from each vertebra can be easily broken, but this may not be particularly painful. If the athlete is unconscious following an injury to the neck, or is complaining about severe neck pain or a tingling or lack of feeling in the limbs, it should be assumed that the neck injury is severe. The neck must be immobilized until x-rays or other evaluations can be made which can rule out any fractures.

An athlete who has had a neck injury should not return to the sport until there are no symptoms and the strength of the neck (forward, backward and sideways) is at least as developed as it was before the injury.

LESS SERIOUS NECK PROBLEMS

Stiff Neck

A stiff neck, or *torticollis,* may be caused by holding the head at an unusual angle, often when sleeping. A nerve or the lining of a neck joint may be pinched, leading to mus-

cle spasm and pain. To relieve this condition, apply a warm compress and gently massage and stretch the neck.

Sprains and Strains

A sprained or strained neck, or 'whiplash' injury, can be caused by a strong force snapping the neck forwards or back. Contact sports and car accidents are the most common causes. Use the standard treatment for relief. A neck collar or brace may be advised, to limit additional injury and minimize the movement that might cause pain.

Pinched Nerve

A pinched nerve or 'burner' occurs when a nerve is pinched or otherwise injured. A quick sideways twist of the neck is the most likely cause. A burning pain can be felt in the neck and usually down the arm. (The nerves that control the arms and hands originate in the neck.) Use the standard treatment.

THE BACK

The Lumbar Spine

Spine-related problems make up about 10 per cent of all athletes' complaints, and back pain is at least a minor problem for three-quarters of all top athletes. The curve and shape of the spine can pre-dispose to back pain, but most problems are due to over-use, with poor muscle control or trauma.

Injuries due to immediate trauma, such as a blow to the back, a fall, or a muscle strain while lifting, are obvious. The problems or causes of over-use injuries are not quite so easily pinpointed. The repetitive small injuries which result in over-use problems can be caused by continued bending forwards or backwards, continued quick or strenuous muscle contractions, or by the continued use of vertebral joints which have degenerated or are arthritic. If pain has persisted for a month to six weeks, it can be considered to be chronic, calling for medical diagnosis and treatment.

Fractures

An immediate fracture can result from a sharp blow to the vertebrae, a strong contraction of the back muscles, or a fall. The pain will be localized, but may radiate down the buttocks and legs, depending on which vertebra was fractured

Stress fractures of the spine *(spondylolysis)* are a serious problem in sports where the back is repeatedly hyper-extended (bent backwards). This movement is common in gymnastics, figure skating, volleyball, football and dance (ballet, modern and jazz). If this occurs on both sides of the back, then one vertebra can slip forward on the other *(spondylolisthesis)*.

LOWER-BACK PROBLEMS

Degenerating Discs

Degenerating discs are a major lower-back problem. Discs are thick jelly-filled cartilage-like shock absorbers between each vertebra. Problems occur when the disc slips slightly out of place, or the jelly-like material inside moves out of its casing. If the bulging disc puts pressure on the nerves in the area, pain may be felt in the lower back and radiate to the buttocks and down the leg(s), often with

pins and needles (for example, sciatica). This pain occurs because the nerves of the buttocks and legs originate between the vertebrae in the area of the lower back. A degenerated disc that does not press on a nerve may or may not cause a local lower-back pain.

Degenerating discs have been found in athletes as young as 10 years. Studies have shown that nearly half of adult athletes, and 11 per cent of athletes under 18 have such disc-related problems. The contributing factors include: a family history of degenerative discs; strenuous lifting (particularly in a lift such as the dead lift, where the torso is at a 90-degree angle and the maximum effort in the lift is done at this point); some collision sports such as American football and rugby. The exaggerated hyper-extended posture of female gymnasts can also place strain on the back side of the discs. Heavy weight-training should be avoided until full maturity, and scrupulous attention must be paid to technique.

Continual forward flexing can cause similar problems, damaging the forward part of the discs. Sports such as rowing, competitive diving, and gymnastics, as well as many forms of dance, can increase the likelihood of this type of problem.

Chronic Lower-Back Pain

A number of factors contribute to chronic lower-back pain, including tight buttock and hamstring muscles, tight connective tissue in the lower back, poor abdominal strength, poor posture ('sway back'), and muscle strains.

Lifting incorrectly can bring on and continue lower-back pain, while American football, gymnastics, wrestling, rowing and tennis are among the sports which are also likely to cause it. Fifty per cent of male Olympic rowers miss training or competition in any one year due to back pain, and nearly 40 per cent of male tournament tennis players have missed at least one tournament due to the same problem. In the tennis serve, the back is arched as it twists with great force.

What to do for lower-back pain:
1. use the standard treatment (alternating hot and cold, and rest);
2. a lumbar support belt or strap may reduce pain;
3. the use of non-steroidal anti-inflammatory drugs (such as aspirin) can reduce inflammation and pain;
4. a doctor may prescribe diazepam for up to four days, but muscle-relaxing drugs are not recommended;
5. lying on the back with the knees up can ease the strain on the spine, but bed rest is not recommended;
6. do slow stretching of the low back and hamstrings;
7. strengthen the abdominal muscles.

Treatment and Prevention

Since there can be several causes of lower-back pain, the treatment must fit the problem. If the problem is a tightened fascia in the lower back or tight hamstrings (muscles in the back of the thighs), stretching is wise. If the vertebrae are somewhat out of place, manipulation may be called for. *But,* if the problem is a stress fracture, manipulation would be unwise. If the problem is increased when the lower back is flexed forwards, such as when sitting, a back support can be used when sitting or driving. Relative rest, with flexibility and strengthening exercises that do not cause pain, normally leads to recovery within six weeks.

Many lower-back problems can be avoided or minimized if the athlete becomes very flexible in the low back and hamstring areas, and keeps the abdominal muscles strong.

Exercises for the Back

Abdominal curls, pelvic tilt, alternate knee to chest, back and hamstring stretches.

CHAPTER 9

The Head and Face

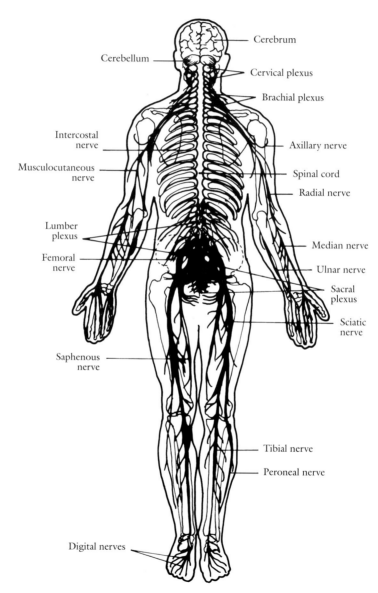

Cerebrum

Cerebellum

Cervical plexus

Brachial plexus

Intercostal
nerve

Axillary nerve

Musculocutaneous
nerve

Spinal cord

Radial nerve

Lumber
plexus

Median nerve

Femoral
nerve

Ulnar nerve

Sacral
plexus

Sciatic
nerve

Saphenous
nerve

Tibial nerve

Peroneal nerve

Digital nerves

Fig 59. The nervous system.

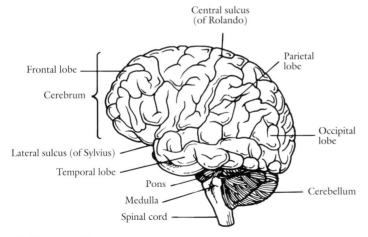

Fig 60. Exterior of brain.

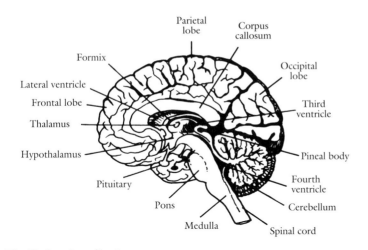

Fig 61. Interior of brain.

THE HEAD

All head injuries must be assumed to be serious by athletes, their coaches, and medical personnel. After a blow to the head, for example, bleeding may occur under the skull from blood vessels on the surface of the brain, and the pressure from the resulting haematoma can be fatal.

Concussion

Concussion is easy to diagnose when the athlete is unconscious, but concussions without unconsciousness are more common. If the athlete cannot remember his or her name, or the type of competition, or shows a lack of alertness, this indicates a concussion. More than 90 per cent of all concussions are of this mild type. However, since even mild concussions can progress to more serious problems, they should be recognized and treated. If there is light-headedness, headache, amnesia, balancing problems, or a lack of feeling in one of the limbs, these must be taken into account as representing a possible head injury.

Medically, concussion is classified as: mild (unconsciousness of up to thirty minutes); moderate (unconsciousness of thirty minutes to a day); or severe (unconsciousness of more than twenty-four hours). Even the mildest form should be adequately treated and the athlete withdrawn from the practice or competition. If an athlete is allowed to return to competition too early there is a danger of 'second

65

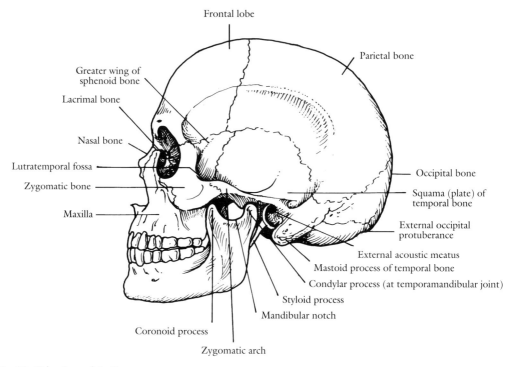

Frontal lobe

Parietal bone

Greater wing of
sphenoid bone

Lacrimal bone

Nasal bone

Lutratemporal fossa

Zygomatic bone

Maxilla

Occipital bone

Squama (plate) of
temporal bone

External occipital
protuberance

External acoustic meatus

Mastoid process of temporal bone

Condylar process (at temporamandibular joint)

Styloid process

Mandibular notch

Coronoid process

Zygomatic arch

Fig 62. Side view of skull.

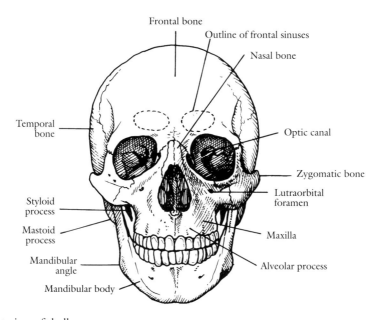

Frontal bone

Outline of frontal sinuses

Nasal bone

Temporal
bone

Optic canal

Zygomatic bone

Lutraorbital
foramen

Styloid
process

Mastoid
process

Maxilla

Mandibular
angle

Alveolar process

Mandibular body

Fig 63. Front view of skull.

---

impact syndrome', in which a second similar concussion is absorbed. This second impact may at first show mild symptoms such as headache, dizziness, or amnesia for up to a minute, then more serious symptoms will develop, including unconsciousness, dilated pupils, and the stopping of breathing.

After a mild (grade 1) concussion, the athlete can return to practice and competition after one week to a month of having no symptoms, depending on the rules of the sport. Symptoms could include headache, dizziness, poor concentration, or memory loss. Most sports have more stringent rules for moderate and severe concussion. Should a second concussion occur, the athlete will have to stay out of competition longer, even for the rest of the season if it is severe. If a third concussion occurs in the same season, then he or she is normally banned from the sport until the next season.

Skull Fracture

A skull fracture can be an extremely serious type of head injury, as the broken skull bones can penetrate the brain and cause additional injury.

Helmets

Helmets like those used in American football, ice hockey, bobsleigh, motor-cycling, bicycle riding and ski competitions can greatly reduce the incidence of skull fracture and concussion. Helmets like those used in horse riding may reduce the risk of skull fracture, but do not greatly reduce the risk of concussion. They lack the 'air management systems' of modern foams and air-filled sacks that dissipate any blow around the skull. Boxing head-gear, used in amateur fights, is designed more to reduce facial cuts than concussion. The most effective of all the helmets are those used in American football, where both air and foam padding are utilized under a strong plastic shell.

First-Aid and Treatment for Head Injuries

If an athlete is unconscious, it must be assumed that there has been both a head and a neck injury. The neck must be immobilized. Even when the victim is conscious there is sometimes a broken neck or back that has not yet severed the spinal cord. Allowing movement, such as standing or walking, may allow the fractured bone to sever the cord and a permanent paralysis can result from this.

Obviously, head and neck injuries must be treated at an appropriate medical facility. X-rays and scans will be needed to confirm or rule out the severity of the injury.

Headaches

Headaches can be caused by a number of internal or external factors, from psychological to physiological. The stress of anticipating an event, or the relaxation after it, can both cause psychologically-induced headaches. Hard endurance exercise and dehydration can also cause headaches.

A blow to the head is better absorbed if the neck muscles are strong and tensed. The tensed neck transfers some of the force to the lower body, so that it is not only the brain that is absorbing the blow, but the trunk as well. For this reason, strong neck muscles can aid in the reduction of brain injuries, as well as vertebral fractures in the

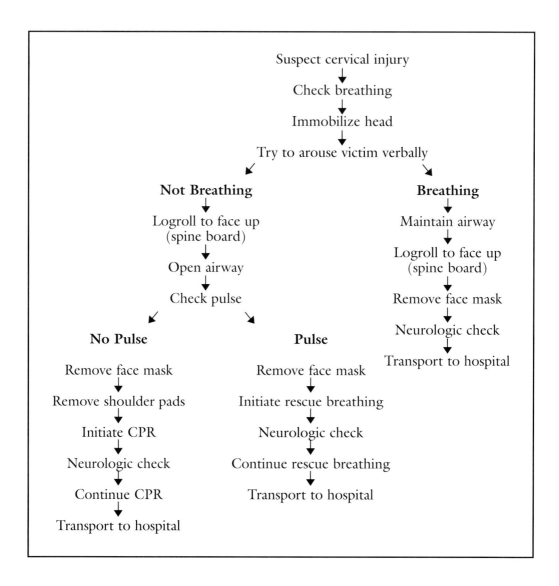

Fig 64. Making decisions in the field – head and neck injuries.

neck and the possibility of a severed spinal cord in the neck area, with its attendant paralysis. (*See* Exercises for the Neck, Chapter 8.)

THE FACE

The Teeth

Dental injuries are a very common type of facial injury. They may be as simple as a chipping of the tooth enamel, which can be artificially replaced, or as severe as a tooth being loosened or knocked out. The more serious kind of injury may be accompanied by damage to the nearby bone. When this is the case, immediate care of a dentist or physician is necessary.

A tooth that has been replanted within thirty minutes of the accident has a 95 per cent chance of being permanently replanted successfully, while a tooth that is not re-planted for two hours has only a 5 per cent chance of success. If a tooth is knocked out, reinsert it in its proper place immediately, and keep constant pressure on it until medical help is found.

Dental injuries can be reduced if a proper mouth-guard is used. Boxing, American football, field hockey, ice hockey, and lacrosse are all sports in which mouth-guards should be used.

Dislocation of the Jaw

Jaw dislocation can be caused by a blow to the jaw or by an action as simple as yawning, sneezing, or yelling. Any action that opens the mouth wide can dislocate the jaw. It can generally be dealt with by putting the thumbs on the top of the back teeth of the jaw, then pressing down and backwards until the jaw is back in place. Once the jaw has been dislocated it is likely to happen again, because the ligaments holding the jaw in place will have been stretched by the initial dislocation, and will not be able to hold the jaw in place as efficiently as before.

THE EARS

The ears can be a particular problem for some athletes. 'Swimmer's ear' (*Otitis externa*) is an inflammation of the ear canal outside the ear drum. Continued wetness in the outer part of the ear can encourage the growth of bacteria, which can set up an infection. Mild cases can be treated with ear drops bought over the counter. More severe cases need to be treated with prescription drugs.

'Cauliflower ear' was once common among wrestlers, before they began wearing ear protectors, and is still seen among boxers. A hit or continued rubbing can cause a separation between the ear cartilage, which forms the ear structure, and the skin. Blood clots in the resulting space, and scar tissue, develop, and this enlarges and deforms the ear.

THE EYES

The eyes are often irritated by foreign bodies such as small insects, or pieces of soot or dust. Sometimes, the resulting tears will bring the foreign body to the inner corner of the eye.

If the object is under the upper eyelid, the upper eyelid can be brought over the lower lid. Often, the object will stick to the lower lid when the upper lid slides back into place. If that doesn't work, roll the upper lid over a cotton swab, a clean pencil or a match stick.

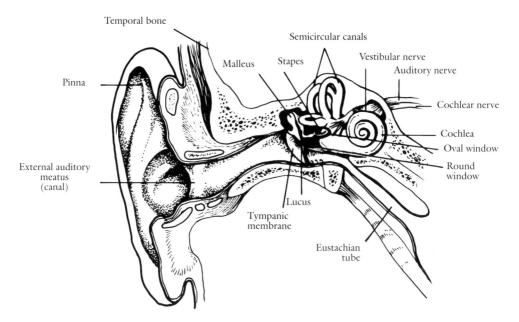

Temporal bone

Semicircular canals

Malleus Stapes

Vestibular nerve

Auditory nerve

Pinna

Cochlear nerve

Cochlea
Oval window

External auditory
meatus
(canal)

Round
window

Lucus

Tympanic
membrane

Eustachian
tube

Fig 65. Interior view of the ear.

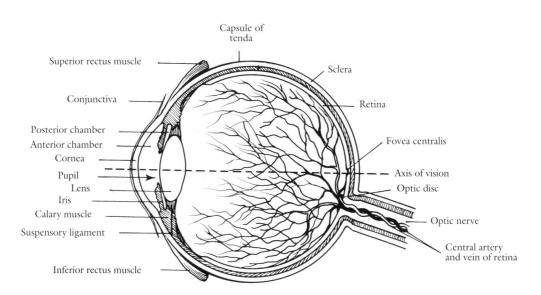

Capsule of
tenda

Superior rectus muscle

Sclera

Conjunctiva

Retina

Posterior chamber
Anterior chamber
Cornea
Pupil
Lens
Iris
Calary muscle
Suspensory ligament

Fovea centralis

Axis of vision
Optic disc

Optic nerve

Inferior rectus muscle

Central artery
and vein of retina

Fig 66. The eye.

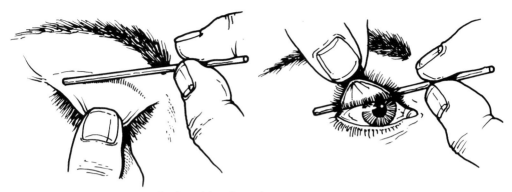

Fig 67. Preparing to remove a foreign object from the eye.

When the object is spotted, use a dampened swab or clean piece of cloth to pick it up. If an object has penetrated the eye ball, or scratched the surface of the eye, seek medical attention.

A blow to the eye can bruise the area around the eye and cause a 'black eye'. The blow to the area bruises the tissues and causes some bleeding under the skin. A cold compress can reduce the blood flow and slow the swelling. Use the standard treatment, as for bruises in any part of the body.

A squash ball is exactly the right size to enter the eye socket and can cause severe injury, so eye protectors should always be worn.

THE NOSE

A nose bleed is the most common type of bleeding condition in sport. It can occur because of a blow to the nose, or because of the dryness of the air, which reduces the nasal mucus and exposes the sensitive membranes. As with most bleeding problems, use cold applications (ice, or a cold wet cloth), and keep the head higher than the rest of the body. Don't lie down. Apply pressure by gently gripping the two nostrils between the thumb and index finger and holding for at least two minutes. When the pressure is released, you should not sniff or blow the nose, as this may loosen the blood clot, causing the bleeding to begin again

A broken nose is not uncommon in contact sports, especially basketball, rugby, football and boxing. Generally, it is not a serious injury. The nasal bones are quite small and are located only in the top of the nose. The lower portion of the nose is skin and cartilage. As with any broken bone, a doctor should be consulted, but a broken nose may not keep the sportsman out of competition. It is quite common to put a padded metal protector over the nose, or use a face mask, and re-enter competition in a day or so.

SUNBURN

Sunburn may be the most harmful skin injury, and the face may be particularly vulnerable. The sun represents a dangerous threat in the development of skin cancers – both benign and malignant. Any sportsperson taking part in outdoor sports – especially skiing – should use a high-factor sun block at all times, and should wear a hat if the weather is sunny.

CHAPTER 10
The Arm

THE UPPER ARM

Fractures of the middle of the upper arm *(humerus)* happen in many sports. The bone can be broken by a direct blow or as a result of over-use, especially in throwing sports. Treatment requires a cast and rest for ten to twelve weeks. This type of fracture may be accompanied by nerve damage and/or blood vessel injury.

Pain or tingling in the upper arm, possibly into the hand and fingers, may be caused by problems with the nerves as they leave the upper spine and neck. Sometimes this is caused by muscle spasms. Heat might help to relax the muscle if spasm is a cause. Sometimes the cause is poor posture, and correcting this can reduce the pain.

Muscle pulls or strains are most likely to occur in the biceps with weight-lifters and in

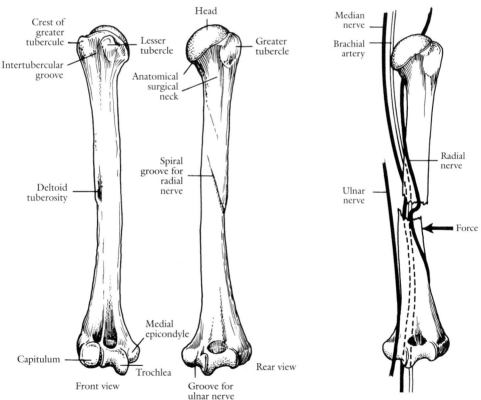

Fig 68. Right humerus (upper arm).

Fig 69. Fracture, with possible nerve damage.

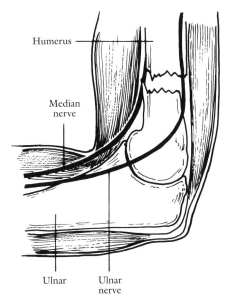

Humerus

Median
nerve

Ulnar   Ulnar
nerve

Fig 70. Break in lower humerus.

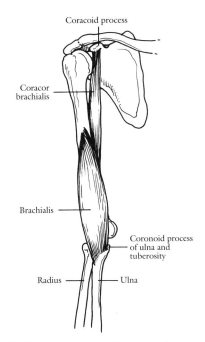

Coracoid process

Coracor
brachialis

Brachialis

Coronoid process
of ulna and
tuberosity

Radius   Ulna

Fig 71. Front upper arm, deep muscles.

the triceps with throwers. The pain is usually sharp, like the stabbing of a knife, rather than dull and more diffuse. Ice and compression are needed immediately. Any contracting of the muscle can reduce the chances of an early cure. A complete rupture of the bicep leads to an obvious lump appearing when contraction is attempted.

Pain in the upper arm, near the shoulder, is likely to be a tendinitis in the biceps tendon or rotator cuff muscles of the shoulder, near where it crosses the top of the upper arm bone. Pushing the thumb deep into the shoulder muscle will generally confirm the area of inflammation, and pain is often felt here on trying to move the arm against resistance.

THE ELBOW

Elbow injuries can occur with a single trauma, a series of stresses, which weakens the elbow, or a lesser single trauma to an already

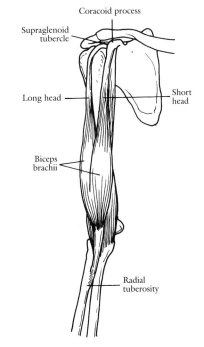

Coracoid process

Supraglenoid
tubercle

Long head

Short
head

Biceps
brachii

Radial
tuberosity

Fig 72. Front upper arm, exterior muscles.

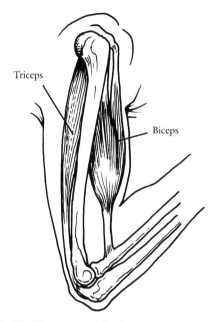

Triceps

Biceps

Fig 73. Upper arm, side view.

weakened elbow that has previously absorbed stresses. The single trauma may be a fall, or a force to the elbow – for example, the arm caught between other players' bodies while tackling in American football or rugby.

'Tennis Elbow' and 'Golfer's Elbow'

The chronically stressed elbow can have muscular, tendon or bursa damage, and pain where the tendon joins the bone on the outside of the elbow is seen in 'tennis elbow'.

'Tennis elbow' *(lateral humeral epicondylitis)* can affect anyone who continually uses the forearm muscles (for example, in gripping a racket). The muscles in the back of the forearm are not as strong as those on the inner side of the forearm, so they are more likely to be injured. Nevertheless, a similar problem can occur on the inside of the elbow; this is called 'golfer's elbow',

although golfers actually suffer more frequently from tennis elbow!

These two problems are more likely to occur if the player is gripping the racket or club too hard, due to inexperience, fatigue or too small a handle. Tennis elbow problems occur in over 40 per cent of recreational tennis players over 30. Vibrations from the racket cause stress to the forearm muscles and the elbow. The further from the middle of the racket that the ball is hit, the more vibrations are developed, so the beginner is much more likely to experience elbow problems in tennis. Their muscles are not conditioned to the sport and their co-ordination is not yet good enough to hit the ball in the middle of the racket on every stroke.

What to do:
1. R.I.C.E.;
2. wear an elbow brace specifically designed for the condition. Most sporting goods stores and tennis shops stock them;
3. to prevent a re-occurrence, or to prevent it from happening in the first place, stretch the wrist and forearm muscles regularly both up and down.

Tendon and muscle problems in the elbow can be prevented if the muscles around the elbow are strengthened and conditioned so that they are able to tolerate more use. For example, to prevent a tennis elbow, do reverse wrist curls, or just grasp the end of a broom and, with the palm facing downwards, lift the broom using only the movement of the wrist. Do this several times each day to strengthen the muscles on the back side of the forearm. This strengthens the arm for backhand drives.

In golfers, elbow problems occur on the inside of the forearm. To prevent this, lift the broom with the palm of the hand facing upwards. Use only a wrist movement. This will also help tennis players to develop more strength for the serve.

'Pitcher's Elbow'

'Pitcher's elbow' *(osteochondritis dissecans)* can be caused by the tearing off of a small chip of bone to which a part of the tendon attaches. In addition to the pain involved, it may result in a locking of the elbow joint. Generally, the athlete will feel pain in the area for some time before the bone is actually fractured.

'Little League Elbow'

'Little League elbow' is the name for damage done to the inside top of the arm bone *(ulna)* just below the elbow. In children this bone is not yet hardened, so it is easily injured. The cartilage is also often injured. The snapping down of the elbow – the action used in pitching a 'curve ball' in baseball – is the major cause, and rest from throwing is needed.

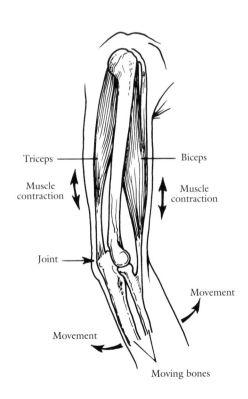

Fig 74. Action of the elbow.

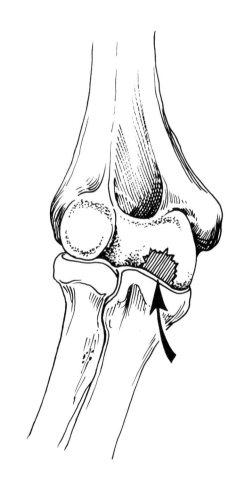

Fig 75. Bone chip missing from elbow.

As with other injuries, use the standard approach of ice, heat, compression, and NSAIDs. Surgery is sometimes called for, but strengthening the area for either prevention or rehabilitation is essential.

The Back of the Elbow

Pain in the back of the elbow often happens when the elbow is straightened further than normal (hyper-extension). It can also happen when something hits the elbow, or when the sportsperson hits something forcefully with the arm straight. The cause of the pain can be a bruise where the top of the main bone of the lower arm (ulna) stops the extension of the arm. The 'hook-like' upper end on the ulna, which moves into a hole in the upper arm bone (humerus), acts like a hammer. The cause of the pain could also be a sprained ligament, inflamed bursa or a strained or inflamed tendon in that area.

What to do:
1. R.I.C.E.;
2. restrict the capacity of the arm to extend;
3. use a sling if pain does not allow the arm to be held normally.

THE FOREARM

Forearm fractures are quite common when a direct blow has occurred. Either of the bones of the lower arm can be fractured. The ulna is the major bone connecting the elbow to the wrist. The *radius* moves around the ulna, allowing turning of the wrist and hand.

Hockey, lacrosse, the martial arts and American football are sports where this kind of fracture is most likely to occur. Extreme displaced fractures are more likely in cycling, motor-racing and motocross. Stress fractures are more likely in racket sports, pitching in baseball, and cricket bowling.

BRUISES

Bruises can occur on any part of the arm in a number of sports in which another person's body or a ball comes into contact with the arm. Ice is the best way to reduce the blood flow and the resulting discoloration.

EXERCISES FOR THE ARMS

Biceps and triceps stretching, curls and extensions, push-ups, tennis ball squeezing, broom lifts, manual resistance.

CHAPTER 11
The Wrist, Hand and Fingers

THE WRIST

The wrist is a very delicate and easily injured joint. With the two forearm bones meeting the wrist and eight bones in the wrist leading to the five bones in the palm of the hand there is a large number of ligaments and joints, all of which can be injured by wrist movements or falls.

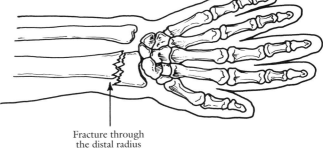

Fracture through the distal radius

Fig 76. Wrist fracture.

The wrist can be injured when the hand is outstretched to break a fall. Over-use wrist injuries are most likely to occur in gymnastics, weight-lifting, or racket sports such as tennis. Hand injuries are more likely to occur in ball-handling sports such as volleyball, baseball, basketball, team handball, and contact sports such as rugby and judo.

Hand and wrist over-use injuries affect 75 per cent of climbers. Hand and wrist injuries are more common in children and youths than in adults.

Fractures

Fractures to the wrist and hand bones can result from a sudden trauma or from repeated stresses, developing a stress fracture. Golfers, tennis players and baseball players are most likely to develop these stress fractures.

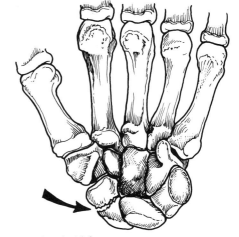

Fig 77. Scaphoid fracture.

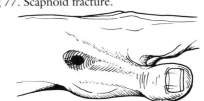

Fig 78. Tenderness with scaphoid fracture.

The bones of the lower arm are called the ulna and the radius. Breaks of the radius near the wrist are quite common, and account for over 10 per cent of all bone injuries commonly seen in athletes. Falls are a common cause of this injury.

The small wrist bone just above the thumb (the *scaphoid*) is commonly the subject of a fracture when the hand is used to break a fall. There will be bony tenderness between the two tendons at the base of the thumb on the inside of the wrist. It is very important not to miss this fracture, since the wrist must be put in plaster immediately or the break will not heal.

Sprains

Wrist sprains are very common. They may accompany a fracture, but they are more commonly experienced without a fracture. Use the standard treatment of ice and heat along with compression, using an elastic wristband or an elastic wrap. Taping around the wrist or using a wrist brace should reduce the chances of an immediate re-occurrence.

If the sprain resulted from a backward bending of the hand, several strips of tape can be used on the inside of the arm and hand. The hand should be bent forwards before the tape is applied. (The degree of forward bend is determined by the amount of backward extension that you feel to be maximal.) Anchor the strips of tape with tape around the hand and around the lower forearm. If the sprain was caused by an excessive forward bend of the wrist, use the same principles, but use the several strips of tape on the back of the hand and wrist.

Over-Use

Over-use injuries to the wrist *(tenosynovitis)* are most likely to occur in golfers, racket-sports players and fly-fishers. The left thumb

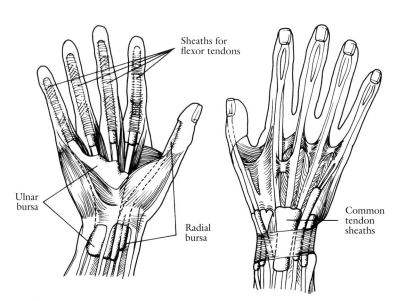

Fig 79. Tendon sheaths of the hand: top (r) and bottom views.

of the right-handed golfer is particularly vulnerable because the wrist is bent far backwards in the backswing.

Carpal and Ulnar Tunnel Syndrome

Carpal tunnel syndrome (common) or ulnar tunnel syndrome (rare) are caused when the nerves which pass the wrist are compressed in one of the tunnels through which they must pass. Carpal tunnel syndrome often occurs with people who use their wrists a good deal in their work, especially in typing or assembling, and is more likely to affect a pregnant woman. It is characterized by pain in the wrist and often by tingling in the thumb and the next two or three fingers. The tingling results when the nerve impulse is disturbed. The ulnar tunnel syndrome will affect the little finger and the ring finger.

What to do:
1. R.I.C.E.;
2. shaking the wrist may loosen the pinching on the nerve;

3. avoid as much as possible bending the wrist forwards. A commercial brace should be helpful.

'Handlebar Palsy'

'Handlebar palsy' *(ulnar neuropathy)* is due to compression and irritation of the nerve on the outside of the hand at the base of the little finger. Gripping the handlebar of a bicycle for long periods of time or leaning on the hands while peddling are the most likely causes. The symptoms include tingling, numbness and weakness. Cyclists can reduce the chances of this happening by changing the position of the hands often while cycling, using padded gloves to absorb the shock, and making certain that the handlebars are not too low. It is important to avoid this condition, or to cure it when it occurs, because permanent damage can result from the continued irritation.

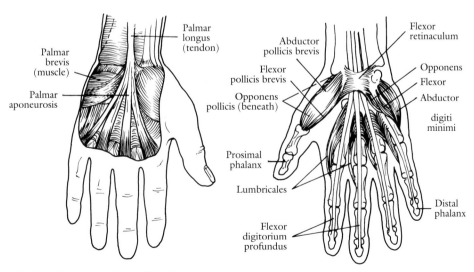

Fig 80. Muscles and tendons of the hand.

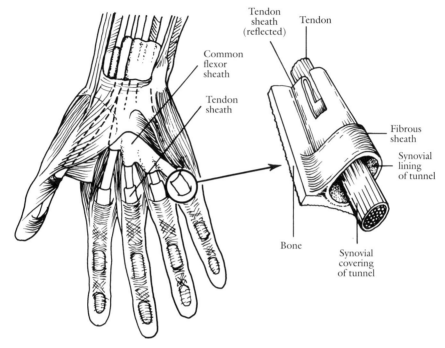

Fig 81. Tendons and sheaths.

Ganglion

A knot in the back of the wrist (*ganglion*) is a lump on a tendon that sometimes follows an injury. The ganglion is due to a weakness in the tendon sheath and will harden when the tendon is tightened. It may be as small as a pea or as big as a grape, and it can be tender. Use ice and compression and protect the lump with a circular pad. It should not limit activities, and often disappears spontaneously, but occasionally a ganglion does need to be removed surgically.

Other Wrist Problems

Wrist problems may occur in athletes whose wrists are bent backwards often during their practice or events. Gymnasts, weight-lifters, golfers and racket-sports players may have

tenderness on the back of the wrist where the wrist bones have been pinched and bruised, or where stress fractures have developed. Gymnastic activities such as walkovers, handstands, vaults, tumbling and balance-beam routines can all cause strains in the wrist.

'Gymnast's wrist' is a premature closing of the bony tissue of the arm bone on the thumb side of the arm (the radius), which stops its growth; it is accompanied by an increased growth of the other bone in the lower arm (the ulna), which then absorbs up to 40 per cent more of the pressure on the hands. A tear in the cartilage-like tissue causes the pain.

'Bugaboo forearm' is a wrist over-use injury suffered by skiers who ski in deep powdery snow. It is caused by the repeated bending backwards of the wrist when withdrawing the pole from deep powder. To reduce the chances of this type of injury, the skier should use poles with smaller baskets, and a shorter pole, and plant the pole less deeply.

For these wrist injuries, use the standard treatment, particularly rest. Injection of cortico-steroids may be carried out by a doctor in order to reduce the inflammation.

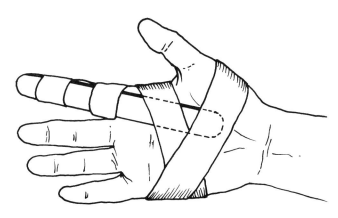

Fig 82. Finger splint.

THE HANDS AND FINGERS

Fractures

Fractures to the hands and fingers are most likely in catching and hitting sports. The fingers can be injured while catching and the hand bones *(metacarpals)* can have compression or stress fractures in hitting sports such as boxing. 'Boxer's fracture' or 'Saturday night fracture' is a break in the hand bone or metacarpal of the little finger, due to the impact of a punch. The pain of a break is usually in the middle of the bone, while the injuries to ligaments are near the joints. Tendon strains can be at any point. If there is any question, see a doctor.

'Mallet Finger'

'Mallet finger' is caused by a rupture of the insertion of a tendon in the back of a finger. The last joint of the finger is affected and the end of the finger cannot be straightened. It is not uncommon in those who play basketball or baseball, and becomes more common as athletes age. The best treatment is generally splinting but sometimes an operation is needed.

Sprains, Dislocations and Jams

Sprains, dislocations and jamming of the fingers are quite common. Athletes in ball sports and in combative sports, such as wrestling and judo, are most susceptible. The dislocation is a more serious type of ligament injury than a sprain or a jam. 'Boxer's knuckle' is a tear in the tendon of the third knuckle – the knuckle most likely to absorb the greatest amount of force in a punch.

The standard treatment of ice, compression and, later, heat, along with movement of the joint, can reduce the swelling in this type of injury. Splinting or taping the finger to an adjacent finger ('neighbour strapping') can reduce the chance of re-injury.

THE THUMB

The thumb can be subject to the same types of injuries, especially when it is bent back when grasping an opponent (as in American football or wrestling), or falling while holding a racket or ski pole. Sprains may range

81

from slight to severe. A complete tear of the ligament on the inside of the base of the thumb ('skier's thumb') is a serious injury and must be surgically repaired within days; otherwise, permanent disability can result. If in doubt, the injured person must see a doctor.

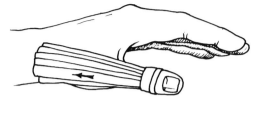

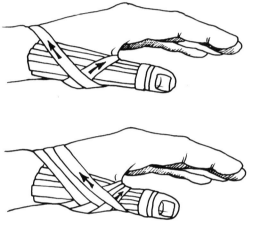

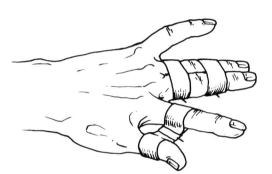

Fig 83. Neighbour strapping.

Fig 84. Taping the thumb.

CHAPTER 12
First Aid

First aid is the immediate and temporary care given to a person who is injured or suddenly taken ill. The first-aider must recognize when it is a serious situation, and give temporary care. In serious cases, this means sustaining the life until the medical specialists arrive and can take over the treatment. The first-aider must make certain to do nothing that will worsen the injury.

First, send for help.

Then, if the injury is life-threatening, think of the A–B–C of first aid:
1. keep the Airway open;
2. maintain the Breathing; and
3. keep the blood Circulating.

When these criteria are not fulfilled, the trained person must consider cardio-pulmonary resuscitation.

BREATHING

Sometimes, the tongue falls against the back of the mouth, such as in a seizure or in a drowning. To alleviate this condition, the victim's head should be gently tilted backwards, with two fingers under the chin. The tongue is a muscle attached to the lower jaw with a heavy tendon that goes to the back of the jaw. Tilting the head will get the tongue off the back of the throat, opening the airway. Check for breathing by looking, listening and feeling: look to see if the chest is rising and falling; listen for air going in and out; and feel the breath. Monitor the breathing to see if the person is breathing at least six times a minute; this is enough to get oxygen into the system and keep the brain alive.

BLOOD CIRCULATION

After evaluating the breathing, the blood circulation must be checked. Place two fingers on the Adam's apple, then draw them towards you, feeling the muscle on the side of the neck. Stick your fingers into the little 'valley' just inside the muscle – this covers the carotid artery – and check for a pulse. Feel for at least thirty seconds, and up to a minute.

If there is a pulse, check to see if the heart is beating at least forty times a minute; this is the number of beats that the average person requires to sustain life by circulating enough blood with oxygen in it to keep the brain alive. If there is inadequate breathing (less than six times a minute) and too low a pulse (below forty beats per minute), then monitor the situation closely. If the breathing and/or pulse stops, mouth-to-mouth resuscitation and/or external compressions (Cardio-Pulmonary Resuscitation, or CPR) should be started. (Everyone dealing with athletes, whether coaches or parents, would be wise to be trained in CPR in case they ever face a situation in which either breathing or circulation stops.)

HIGHEST PRIORITY	SECOND PRIORITY	LOWEST PRIORITY
• Airway and breathing difficulties • Cardiac arrest if sufficient personnel available • Uncontrolled or suspected severe bleeding • Severe medical problems: poisoning, diabetic and cardiac emergencies, etc. • Open chest or abdominal wounds • Shock	• Burns • Major or multiple fractures • Back injuries with or without spinal cord damage	• Fractures or other injuries of a minor nature • Obviously mortal wounds where death appears reasonably certain • Obviously dead • Cardiac arrest (if sufficient personnel are not available to care for numerous other victims) • Follow local protocol

PROCEDURES

1. The most knowledgeable First Aider arriving in the first ambulance must become triage leader.
2. Primary survey should be completed on all victims first. Correct immediate life-threatening problems.
3. Ask for additional assistance if needed.
4. Assign available manpower and equipment to highest priority victims.
5. Arrange for transport of highest priority victims first.
6. If possible, notify emergency personnel and/or hospital(s) of number and severity of injuries.
7. Triage rescuer remains at scene to assign and co-ordinate manpower, supplies and vehicles.
8. Victims must be reassured regularly for changes in condition.

Fig 85. Priorities for First Aid.

CHECKING THE INJURED PERSON

Once breathing and circulation have been established, the whole body should be quickly checked for any type of injury, such as bleeding, which must be stopped as quickly as possible. A person can bleed to death in less than five minutes, and a stopped heart can begin brain death in four to six minutes. Because the time needed to prevent death is so short, the problems have to be identified quickly and the appropriate treatment started.

The Head and Neck

If the person is unconscious and there are no breathing, pulse or bleeding problems, check him or her from head to toe. Beginning at the head, look in each eye,

What is CPR?

Cardio-pulmonary resuscitation (CPR) combines rescue breathing (also known as mouth-to-mouth) and external chest compressions. Cardio refers to the heart and pulmonary refers to the lungs. Resuscitation refers to revival. Proper and prompt CPR serves as a holding action by providing oxygen to the brain and heart until advanced cardiac life support can be provided.

When to start CPR

Trained people need to be able to:
- Recognize the signs of cardiac arrest,
- Provide CPR, and
- Call for emergency medical services.

About two-thirds of deaths that are the result of a heart attack in a non-hospital setting occur within two hours of the first signs and symptoms of a heart attack.

Victims have a good chance of surviving if:
- CPR is started within the first 4 minutes of heart stoppage, and
- They receive advanced cardiac life support within the next 4 minutes.

Brain damage begins within 4–6 minutes after the heart stops and is certain after 10 minutes when no CPR is given.

Start CPR as soon as possible!

Fig 86. Cardio–Pulmonary Resuscitation (CPR).

observing the pupils to see if they react to light or if one is dilated or larger than the other one. This may be an indication that there has been a head or neck injury. If so, the head and neck should be immobilized immediately. This can occur if a blow to the head is received, or if two athletes collide on the field or court.

Next, check for fluid coming from the ears or nose; this could be spinal fluid, which is clear or slightly yellow. If there is blood coming from the nose, but the blood seems to be coming faster or is thinner than normal, this could indicate a skull fracture, with the fluid coming from the spine. Again, the head and neck should be immobilized.

Next, the scalp should be checked. When checking the head or scalp, make sure not to lift the head off the ground because there may have been a neck injury. Don't move the neck. Reach under the neck from the base of the head, through the neck and down to the base of the shoulders. The scalp is checked by running your fingers through the hair to see if there is an open wound, a lump, or a depression. A lump or a depression indicates the trauma received could be sufficiently significant to cause a concussion or a haemorrhage in the brain, and the head and neck should be immobilized immediately. Any bleeding should be treated as described above.

The back of the neck should be checked next. Check for a lump or depression or, if the patient is conscious, some type of pain. A depression or an area that feels like a hole could be a spinal fracture. A lump next to the backbone may indicate a dislocation of a vertebra that could be pinching off the spinal column. In either of these cases, the head and neck should be immobilized immediately.

The Clavicle and Shoulders

The collar bone (clavicle) should be the next area to be examined. Examine one side at a time. Begin by running a finger along the bone from just below the neck, at the top of the ribs, then move your finger slowly along the bone and out towards the shoulders. If the bone does not seem smooth, there may be a fracture. Determining whether or not there is a fracture of either or both of the collar bones will help decide how the athlete may be lifted for transport. If there is a fracture, the athlete should not be lifted by the shoulders, as this could lead to a compound fracture.

The Ribs and Abdomen

The ribs need to be looked at next. Place both hands on both sides of the ribs, just under the arms, about half-way down the ribs, and gently press in, without lifting the athlete off the ground. If there is pain in the rib area, it is likely that a fracture has occurred. If no pain is felt during the first test, place the heel or side of the hand on the sternum and push down once to move the ribs to see if there is pain and a possible fracture.

Next, check the abdominal area. Using the flat of your fingers, start at the ribs and press gently several times, moving your hand in a counter-clockwise direction. Start just under the ribs on the athlete's right side, going down to the hip bone, across the lower abdomen, back up into the rib cage, and then back to the middle starting point. In doing this, you are checking for a hard rigid spot, which would indicate gross bleeding inside the abdominal area. If this occurs, it is a definite medical emergency. If you find a tender area, it would indicate that the trauma experienced has broken blood vessels. If this is not treated immediately and properly, it could turn to a hard rigid area, and the athlete could bleed to death. In this situation, the athlete should be immobilized on a spine board, if possible, not allowed to get up and move around, and taken to a doctor as soon as possible for the appropriate treatment.

The Back and Spine

The low back should be checked next. Place your hand on the spine in the lower back, and feel the curvature. As with the upper back, feel for a lump or a depression. A lump would indicate a dislocation of a vertebra from the lower back, which could cause paralysis or a lack of sensation to the legs. A depression could indicate a fracture and show that a part of a vertebra is pushed in on the spinal column. Immobilization on a spine board would be the course of action.

The Pelvic Area

To check the pelvic area, place your hands on either side of the legs where they attach to the hips. Push in and gently lift up, not actually lifting the body off the ground, but moving the bones slightly. If the athlete has incurred a fracture to the pelvic bone(s), getting up and walking could cause the bones to slide past one another, and sharp bones could cut the intestines and cause an infection inside the body. Such an infection is extremely difficult to cure.

The Arms

Now check the arms. Place your hand on the arm nearest to you. Put one hand under the shoulder, the other hand under the upper arm and, with firm hard pressure, feel the arm all the way down to the elbow, and from the elbow to the wrist. Ask the injured person to squeeze your index and middle fingers hard enough to show control. Now go to the other arm, following the same procedure. If the athlete cannot squeeze, or there is no control of the arms, this indicates a possible neck injury, with the control of the arm not being relayed from the brain through the neck down into the muscles. In this case, immobilization is indicated.

The Legs

Next, examine the legs by compressing the muscles of the thigh around the femur, all the way along to the knee, and from the knee to the ankle. Place your hand on the bottom of the foot and ask the athlete to move the foot against the pressure you are gently applying. Be sure that the athlete knows which foot you are asking him or her to use, as you may be led wrongly to assume that the athlete is paralysed. Follow these same steps on the other leg. If the athlete is unable to move either foot, or there is no sensation in that leg, a lower back injury

may have occurred. Immobilization on a spine board is indicated, with immediate emergency treatment to rule out a spinal injury by proper medical personnel.

REHABILITATION

Athletes need to be treated early for their injuries, but they must also keep their muscle strength up so that they can return quickly to competition. Muscle strength may be reduced by as much as 17 per cent within the first three days after injury. The loss of strength over the next several days is less rapid, but strength losses of up to 40 per cent may occur while an arm or leg is in a cast for six weeks. If you cannot continue your strength training in the injured area, it is important to continue to train the uninjured areas of your body.

Aerobic fitness is also reduced quickly. The VO2 max (the measure of aerobic fitness used for top-level athletes) reduces by up to 25 per cent if the athlete is forced to rest in bed for three weeks. Consequently, if your injury allows you to continue to train in another activity, do it. If you have an injury to your foot, try swimming or cycling. If you are a swimmer with 'swimmer's shoulder', you can run or cycle.

WOUNDS

An abrasion is the most common kind of wound. In an abrasion the first two or three layers of the skin are scraped off and there is minimal bleeding. Other types of wounds are incisions or lacerations. An incision is a smooth cut, while a laceration is a jagged cut which sometimes pierces the skin and cuts into the soft tissue below, and possibly even

Incision

Avulsion

Puncture

Abrasion

Laceration

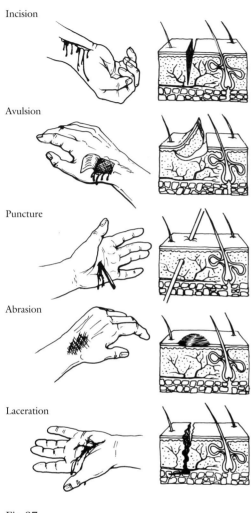

Fig 87

Ointment

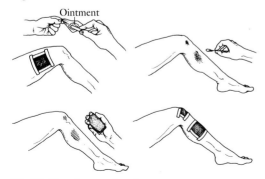

Fig 88. Treating an abrasion.

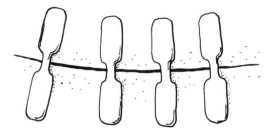

Fig 89. Butterfly taping of a cut.

into the muscle tissue. In such cases there would be more bleeding, often very severe.

Other types of wound are: a puncture, where the skin is pierced down into other soft tissue; usually, when the object is removed, the injury will seal and have minimal bleeding, but care is needed to make sure no foreign body is left in the hole; an avulsion, where a piece of the tissue is torn away; an amputation, where an appendage of the body, such as the end of a finger, a hand or a foot, is cut off.

BLEEDING

Direct Pressure

The first aid procedure for bleeding is to put direct pressure on the wound; even when there is an amputation, where a portion of the body has been severed, direct pressure is the first approach. In skiing, fingers and hands have been amputated by being run over with the sharp edge of a ski. In a case such as this, that direct pressure could be as simple as an index finger and thumb reaching in and pinching the artery that has been severed. However, direct pressure normally means compressing the capillaries in the skin or just under the skin, using your hand. It is best to have a clean cloth between your hand and the wound; this could be the kind

Type	Symptoms and Nature	Emergency Care
Capillary	Oozing, most common type of external haemorrage. This type of bleeding is expected in all minor cuts, scratches, and abrasions. Dark bluish-red colour.	External bleeding is bleeding that can be seen coming from a wound. Excessive external bleeding can create a crisis situation: the platelets, which usually help the blood clot, aren't effective in cases of severe bleeding or when the blood vessels have been damaged. Serious blood loss is defined as 2 pints (1 litre) in an adult and 1 pint (0.5 litre) in a child. If the bleeding remains uncontrolled, shock and death may result. **Elevate Extremity** **Direct Pressure** 1. Apply direct pressure against the bleeding site. 2. Use a dressing; if necessary, even your bare hand. If dressing soaks through do not remove it; put another on top and continue applying pressure. 3. Maintain firm pressure until the bleeding stops or until the patient reaches the hospital. 4. If the wound is an extremity, elevate it while you apply direct pressure. **Pressure Points** The most important arteries used in pressure point control include: **The brachial artery,** along the inside of the upper arm midway between the elbow and the shoulder; compression will stop or control bleeding below the pressure point. **The femoral artery,** in the groin, slows bleeding in the leg on the appropriate side.
Venous	Slow, even blood flow. Occurs when a vein is punctured or severed. Venous blood is dark in colour (maroon). Danger in venous bleeding from neck wound is that an air bubble may be sucked into the wound.	
Arterial	Occurs when an artery is punctured or severed. Not common because arteries are located deep in the body and are protected by bones. Arterial bleeding is characterized by spurting of bright red blood. Common arteries injured in accidents: carotid, brachial, radial, femoral.	

Splints

In cases of open fractures, splintered bone ends can damage tissue and cause external bleeding. Properly applied splints can immobilize the fracture and lessen the chance of further injury.

Tourniquet

Use of a tourniquet is rarely warranted, because control of external bleeding can almost always be achieved by using some other means. Tourniquets should be used as a last resort only, and only after trying all other methods of control.

Fig 90. Treatments for external bleeding.

of sterile dressing, such as a gauze pad, commonly found in first aid kits, or any type of clean absorbent cloth.

Direct pressure should be applied for at least three to five minutes, or until the bleeding has stopped. In order to hold the dressing on with the proper pressure, a pressure bandage should be used. This may be a roller gauze bandage, a triangular bandage, or some type of material that can be made to put pressure on the wound by tying it tightly to the body. You can add more gauze pads to the wound to absorb the increased blood flow. As a secondary measure, elevation of the bleeding body part above the heart for five minutes will also help.

Symptoms	Cause
Bright red frothy blood coughed up indicates bleeding in the lungs. Fast and shallow breathing, rapid weak pulse, moist skin.	Punctured lungs from broken ribs.
Vomiting bright red blood.	Bleeding in stomach.
Vomiting dark brown (coffee ground-like) blood.	Older blood from stomach.
Swelling or discoloration due to a hard blow to any part of the body.	Possible broken bone with internal bleeding.
Black stools or spasm of muscles in the abdominal area.	Appendicitis, intestinal disease
Blood in urine (possibly a smoky colour)	Ruptured bladder, fractured pelvis, kidney injury, urethra injury.

Fig 91. Symptoms and causes of internal bleeding.

Pressure Points

If these measures do not stop the bleeding, and blood continues to seep through the bandages, add more bandages and proceed to the third line of defence – stopping the blood flow by putting pressure on a pressure point higher up on the extremity. The two most likely pressure points to use would be the brachial artery, on the inside of the upper arm between the elbow and the armpit, and the femoral artery, in the inside front of the upper leg where the leg attaches to the hip.

Putting direct pressure on an artery, and pushing it against the bone nearest the artery, will pinch off the flow of blood from the heart to that extremity, helping to stop

the bleeding. If the pressure point is held for approximately five minutes, the bleeding will usually stop because the blood at the site of the wound should have had a chance to coagulate.

Any place on the body where a pulse is felt may be used as a pressure point. The radial pulse is on the thumb side of the wrist; applying pressure here should stop the bleeding on the palm side of the hand and the thumb. If bleeding is on the back of the hand, or the fingers, the ulnar pulse is used; it is on the same side of the wrist as the little finger. The pulse located behind the knee, when pressed, should stop bleeding in the lower leg. The foot has a pulse behind the ankle bone on the inside, or medial side, just behind the lower-leg bone (the *tibia*). There

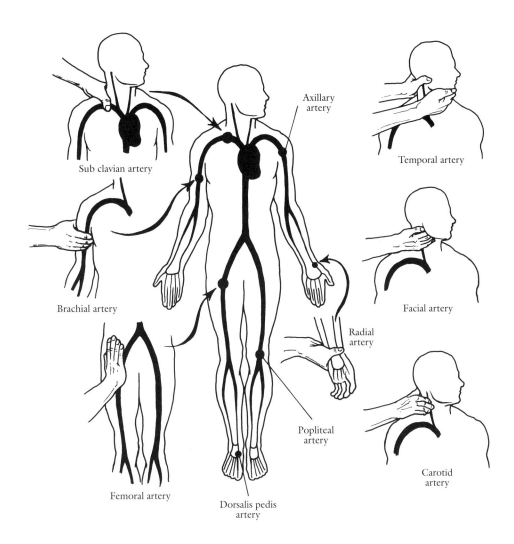

Sub clavian artery

Axillary artery

Temporal artery

Brachial artery

Facial artery

Radial artery

Popliteal artery

Carotid artery

Femoral artery

Dorsalis pedis artery

Fig 92. Pressure points.

is another across the top of the instep where the foot bends and attaches to the leg. There is a pulse on the temporal areas of the head just in front of and above the ears. If there is bleeding on the top of the head, the fore-head, or above the ear, pressure may be applied on the appropriate side of the face at the temporal area.

The Carotid Artery

Most people know that there is a pulse in the carotid artery, located on either side of the Adam's apple. This should *not* be used as a pressure point to stop bleeding in the head; such a measure would stop blood flow to the brain.

FRACTURES

Bones are sometimes broken during sporting activities, and it is important to know what first– aid measures to take. The point of the break should be immobilized by splinting – attaching a rigid implement from above the joint to below it. The immediate goal is to immobilize the two broken bone ends and the joints above and below them. Never attempt to straighten, pull, or set the broken bone ends, as this may lead to further injury to blood vessels or nerves. Once the splinting has taken place, take the injured person to the doctor, who may apply a cast so that healing can take place during the next four to six weeks.

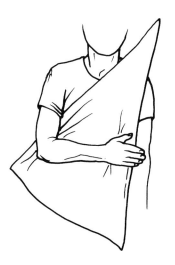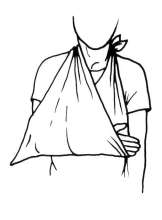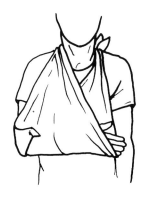

Fig 93 Making a sling

CHAPTER 13

Environmental Problems

There are a number of external factors that can increase the risk of injury to an athlete. Incorrect or inadequate protective equipment for ice hockey or American football players, or a poor surface on the field of play are obvious examples, but the temperature, the level of humidity, and air pollution can contribute just as much to the risk of serious injury.

HEAT

Excess heat not only negatively affects performance but it also can be a source of seri-ous health problems. As the outside temper-ature increases, it becomes less and less pos-sible to get rid of the heat of the body produced by exercise. For example, a person exercising at 37 degrees Fahrenheit (3 degrees centigrade) is 20 per cent more effective in eliminating body heat than someone exercising at 78 degrees Fahrenheit (20 degrees centigrade), and 150 per cent more effective than someone exercising at 104 degrees Fahrenheit (40 degrees centi-grade). Normal resting body temperature is 98.6 degrees Fahrenheit (37 degrees centi-grade), but it is not uncommon for the body to reach a temperature of 104 to 105

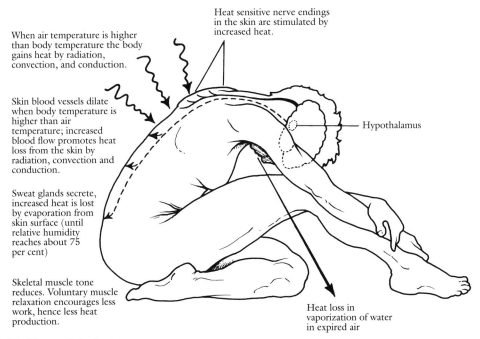

Heat sensitive nerve endings in the skin are stimulated by increased heat.

When air temperature is higher than body temperature the body gains heat by radiation, convection, and conduction.

Skin blood vessels dilate when body temperature is higher than air temperature; increased blood flow promotes heat loss from the skin by radiation, convection and conduction.

Sweat glands secrete, increased heat is lost by evaporation from skin surface (until relative humidity reaches about 75 per cent)

Skeletal muscle tone reduces. Voluntary muscle relaxation encourages less work, hence less heat production.

Hypothalamus

Heat loss in vaporization of water in expired air

Fig 94. Heat and the body.

Air Temperature	0%	10%	20%	30%	40%	50%	60%	70%	80%	90%	100%
120	107	116	130	148							
115	103	111	120	135	151						
110	99	105	112	123	137	150					
105	95	100	105	113	123	135	149				
100	91	95	99	104	110	120	132	144			
95	87	90	93	96	101	107	114	124	136		
90	83	85	87	90	93	96	100	106	113	122	
85	78	80	82	84	86	88	90	93	97	102	108
80	73	75	77	78	79	81	82	85	86	88	91
75	69	70	72	73	74	75	76	77	78	79	80
70	64	65	66	67	68	69	70	70	71	71	72

Apparent Temperature*

Relative Humidity

*Degrees Fahrenheit.
Above 130°F = heat stroke imminent.
105°–130°F = heat exhaustion and heat cramps likely and heat stroke with long exposure and acitivity.
90°–105°F = heat exhaustion and heat cramps with long exposure and activity.
80°–90°F = fatigue during exposure and activity.

Fig 95 Heat Index

degrees Fahrenheit (40 to 41 degrees centigrade) when exercising. High temperature, when combined with high humidity, makes it difficult, or impossible, for perspiration to evaporate so the body can't be cooled effectively. A dry heat is much easier to tolerate, since it allows the sweat to evaporate easily.

The heat generated in the muscles is released by:
1. conduction – from the warmer muscles to the cooler skin;
2. convection – the release of the heat from the skin to the air; and
3. evaporation – the vaporization of the perspiration.

Conduction occurs as the body's liquids, such as the blood, absorb the heat created by the contraction of the muscles and move it to the cooler skin. Water can absorb many thousands of times more heat than air can, so blood is an excellent conductor of heat from the muscles.

Convection occurs when the heat near the skin is absorbed into the atmosphere. For a swimmer in a cool pool, effective convection is very easy. For the runner, it is more difficult. It is aided by a lower air temperature and by wind, which affects the body temperature by cooling it faster than the air temperature would warrant – the 'wind chill factor' experienced on colder days.

Conduction	*Body heat is lost to objects through direct physical contact*
Convection	*Body heat is lost to surrounding air, which becomes warmer, rises, and is replaced with cooler air*
Evaporation	*Body heat causes perspiration which cools the body as it evaporates*
Radiation	*Body heat is lost to nearby objects without physically touching them*

Fig 96. Mechanisms of heat loss from the body.

(See Fig 99.) Even on warmer days, the wind will evaporate perspiration faster and so cool the body more effectively. This may increase the need for fluids, to continue the production of sweat. A four mile an hour wind is twice as effective in cooling as a one mile an hour wind (this is the basis for the wind chill factor).

Evaporation is the most effective method for cooling an exercising body. Each litre (1.75 pints) of sweat that evaporates takes with it 580 kilocalories, or enough heat to raise the temperature of ten litres (17.5 pints) of water by 58 degrees centigrade (137 degrees Fahrenheit). As the skin is cooled by the evaporation of the sweat, it is able to take more of the heat from the blood; cooling the blood allows it to pick up more heat from the muscles.

HUMIDITY

Humidity is the most important factor regulating the evaporation of sweat, which produces the cooling effect as the sweat changes from liquid to gas. Exercising in a rubber suit has a similar effect to exercising in high humidity because the water cannot evaporate. More and more sweat is produced by the body, in a desperate attempt to cool the skin, and the sweat cannot evaporate quickly enough. It drips off the body, and this does not produce the cooling effect that evaporation produces. There is the added danger of dehydration which, if severe, can cause sweating to stop, leading to a very rapid rise in temperature, collapse, and potentially fatal heat stroke.

SALTS AND FLUIDS

The ingredients of sweat change with exercise. Initially, a number of salts are excreted, including sodium chloride (common table salt), potassium, calcium, chromium, zinc, and magnesium salts. As the exercise continues, the amount of salts in the sweat is reduced as some of the body's hormones come into play. Aldosterone, for example, conserves the sodium for the body. Consequently, the longer exercise lasts, the more the sweat resembles pure water.

A normal diet replaces all of the necessary elements lost in sweat. Water alone can be used for fluid replacement, but hypotonic sports drinks (with a lower concentration of salts and sugars than the body) will speed the passage of fluid from the stomach into the small intestine, and so speed absorption. This also provides extra calories during exercise. Sportspeople doing long-distance events in cool environments need sugars more than water; the best drinks are those which contain glucose polymers (maltodextrins). Always check the label on a fluid replacement drink. Caffeine (coffee, tea and cola drinks) and alcohol dehydrate the body, and should be avoided.

Adequate fluid is essential to the functioning of an efficient body. Exercise should be started with the body fully hydrated (the urine should be very pale), and there should be frequent breaks for fluid intake. However, in hot, humid environments, even frequent breaks seldom give an athlete enough fluid. Feeling thirsty indicates 2 per cent dehydration, and athletic performance is affected at more than 1 per cent dehydration, so athletes must be encouraged to drink more water than they think they need. As much as 1.5 litres (2½ pints) of water may be lost before feeling thirsty. A tennis player may lose 0.5–2.5 litres (1–4½ pints) of water in an hour; older athletes, women, and those not accustomed to exercising in heat, are the most vulnerable to dehydration.

ACCLIMATIZATION

Acclimatization is the process by which the body adjusts to a warmer and/or more humid climate. Any sportsperson competing in a humid climate, to which he or she is unaccustomed, will probably take ten days to two weeks to acclimatize properly (Bergeron, M. *et al*, 'Fluid and electrolyte losses during tennis in the heat, *Racquet Sports: Clinics in Sports Medicine,* Vol. 14, 1 Jan 1995). Acclimatization can be quicker in well-trained athletes, who are often partly acclimatized already, and it will be quicker in

anyone who takes regular exercise in the new environment. Tolerance and ability to recover from exercise is reduced until the body is fully acclimatized, and this should be taken into account when planning training or competition schedules.

Among the changes that will probably occur are: an increase in the amount of blood plasma; increased sweating; earlier perspiring; and decreased salt losses. Psychological adjustments will also need to be made to cope with the experience of greater heat and humidity. It is essential to drink large volumes of fluid once acclimatized, as the body will sweat even more than usual.

CLOTHING

The best warm-weather clothing is nothing at all, but this isn't always possible! Changing to dry clothes is not advised because the evaporation effect is maximized when the clothing is wet. Some sports, such as American football, have particular problems with heat. The padding covers nearly 50 per cent of the body, and evaporation cannot take place from those protected areas. Studies have been done on sportspeople performing the same exercise wearing shorts or wearing full American football equipment. There was a difference in rectal temperature between the two of 1.1 degree Fahrenheit (0.6 degrees centigrade) – a maximum of 102.2 degrees Fahrenheit (39 degrees centigrade) for those in the full equipment, and 101.1 degrees Fahrenheit (38.4 degrees centigrade) for those in shorts.

REHYDRATION

While it is recommended that those who exercise should replace 100 per cent of the fluids they lose, this is seldom done. Most will replace only about 50 per cent during the exercise period. Dehydration of 4 per cent of the body's weight will reduce endurance by 30 per cent in temperate conditions, and by as much as 50 per cent when the weather is very warm. Checking weight before and after exercise (unclothed, or in dry clothes) is instructive. Each kilo (2.2lb) of weight lost means the loss of 1 litre (1.75 pints) of water.

Exercise in cold weather also requires adequate fluid intake. The air breathed in needs to be warmed, the body is still producing heat, and there will be a tendency to produce more urine. These factors mean that more fluid must be taken in. If it isn't, the body will feel colder, because the blood will not have sufficient volume to warm the skin effectively with the heat that it picks up from the exercising muscles.

HEAT-RELATED PROBLEMS

To diagnose a heat-related problem, a rectal thermometer should be used; this will give a true temperature, not affected by the cooling effects of sweating and other factors. The temperature during and immediately after exercise should be below 104 degrees Fahrenheit (40 degrees centigrade).

Heat Cramps

Cramping is generally found in the legs, arms or abdomen. The sufferer will be able to think clearly and will have a normal rectal temperature. The treatment is to give fluids with salt, and possibly other minerals (found in most fluid replacement drinks). Heat cramps are particularly common among athletes who are not yet in good physical condition and who are participating in early workouts during warm days. There should be no problem in returning to activity the next day.

Hyperthermia

Hyperthermia, or an excessively high temperature, can develop during exercise, particularly when the sweat cannot evaporate (due to high humidity or excessive clothing). It is a serious complication of dehydration and can lead to heat exhaustion and heat stroke (see page xx). It is possible to lose up to 8 pints (1 to 5 litres) of water during exercise, so dehydration is a very real possibility. The combination of dehydration and a high body temperature can cause a number of physiological problems, including a reduction of blood volume, an increase in the breakdown of liver and muscle glycogen (a sugar used for muscle energy), and the inability of the body to pass certain electrolytes effectively across the cells' membranes.

Heat Exhaustion

Water-depletion heat exhaustion is caused by insufficient water intake and/or excessive sweating. The symptoms may include the following: intense thirst, weakness, chills, fast breathing, impaired judgement, nausea, a lack of muscular co-ordination, and/or dizziness. If untreated it can develop into heat stroke. A rectal temperature of over 104 degrees Fahrenheit (40 degrees centigrade) is the sign. The immediate treatment is to give water or an electrolyte replacement

	Heat Cramps
SIGNS AND SYMPTOMS	1. Severe muscle cramps in arms or legs.
	2. Muscle cramping may occur in the abdominal muscles.
	3. Profuse sweating.
MANAGEMENT OF HEAT CRAMPS	1. Immediate cessation of exercise.
	2. Consumption of fluids, either water or some type of solution containing sodium chloride (table salt) at a concentration of about one teaspoon of salt per 2 pints (1 litre) of water.
	3. Static stretching of the involved muscles.

	Heat Exhaustion
SIGNS AND SYMPTOMS	1. Moist, clammy skin.
	2. Muscle fatigue (general).
	3. Nausea or related gastrointestinal distress.
	4. Dizziness and occasionally loss of consciousness.
	5. Increased respiratory rate and rapid pulse.
	6. Body temperature ranging from 101°F to 104°F (38.5°C to 40°C).
MANAGEMENT OF HEAT EXHAUSTION	1. Immediate cessation of exercise.
	2. Move the athlete to a cool place.
	3. Place the athlete in a supine position, with legs elevated 8–12in (20–30cm).
	4. Loosen clothing and cool the athlete with wet towels or ice packs.
	5. If the athlete is not fully recovered within 30 minutes, seek medical attention.

	Heat Stroke
SIGNS AND SYMPTOMS	1. Sweating may or may not.
	2. Hot, dry skin.
	3. Mental confusion and possible loss of conciousness.
	4. Gastrointestinal distress, including nausea, vomiting and cramping.
	5. Severe motor disturbances and loss of co-ordination.
	6. Rapid and strong pulse.
MANAGEMENT OF HEAT STROKE	1. This is a medical emergency: summon EMS.
	2. Move the athlete to a cool dry place.
	3. Wrap the athlete in wet sheets or towels, or place cold packs in areas with abundant blood supply, e.g., neck, armpits, head and groin.
	4. Treat for shock and monitor temperature. Do not allow body temperature to drop below 102°F (39°C).
	5. Keep the athlete in a semi-seated position.

	Prevention of Heat Disorders
	1. Consume fluids and avoid dehydration when participating in activities in warm and humid environments. Experts recommend the consumption of 0.5 pint (0.25 litres) of water every 30 minutes of activity.
	2. Avoid heavy exertion during times of extreme environmental conditions, especially when the temperature is above 95°F (35°C) and there is high humidity.
	3. Wear proper clothing. Remember that restrictive garments can impair circulation of air, thus reducing the evaporation of sweat. Be aware that dark colours on uniforms and helmets may facilitate heat build-up.
	4. Be reminded that fitness has a positive effect on the ability to function in extreme conditions. The process of developing a tolerance to extremes of climate, or acclimatization, normally requires a period of weeks.

Fig 97. Prevention and management of heat disorders.

drink. A severe case may require intravenous fluid replacement. The skin will generally feel cool and somewhat moist.

Salt-depletion heat exhaustion appears to be similar to heat cramps, and can occur when large volumes of sweat are replaced only with water. If a great deal of salt is lost in the perspiration, this can affect muscle functioning. (Sodium loss is much greater than potassium loss.) It is most likely to occur during the first five to ten days of exercising in the heat. The symptoms may include the following: vomiting, nausea, inability to eat, diarrhoea, a headache (particularly in the front of the head), weakness, a lower body temperature, and muscle cramps. Weight loss and thirst are not symptoms of this problem.

To prevent these heat-related problems, trainers often insist that an athlete must regain 80 per cent of his or her fluid loss before leaving the locker room. If an athlete weighed 165lb (75kg) before the practice and 160lb (73kg) afterwards, the trainer should ask the athlete to take in enough fluids to return to 164lb (74.6kg).

Heat Stroke

Heat stroke can be caused by heavy exercise or by exercising in high temperatures. A very serious condition, which can affect many of the organs, it can occur when the interior organs of the body are heated above 107 degrees Fahrenheit (42 degrees centigrade). At this temperature, the body's protein begins to break down. Enzymes are affected, as are the cell walls. When the cells cannot function effectively, the organ functioning is impaired.

In addition to a body temperature in excess of 104 degrees Fahrenheit (40 degrees centigrade), there can be a rapid pulse (100 to 120 beats per minute), and low blood pressure. There may also be confusion (similar to that experienced after a head injury in contact sports), weakness, fatigue, or delirium; the victim can lapse into a coma. There may or may not be sweating. The pupils of the eyes may be very small.

When the problem is caused by physical exertion, the skin will probably be an ashen colour, indicating poor circulation. When it is caused solely by the sun, or by general over-heating, the skin is more likely to be red.

Treatment should be immediate, aiming to cool the body, and bring about effective rehydration; this often has to be intravenous. Don't wait for the hospital to treat the victim; it may be too late. Use ice packs to the neck, and groin. Full immersion in a bath of cold water is better. You can also spray with a hose. Once the temperature returns to 100 to 101 degree Fahrenheit (38 or 39 degrees centigrade), the cooling process should be slowed.

At competitions where heat stroke is a possibility, tubs, whirlpools or inflatable boats filled with cold water are a wise preparation. Anyone who has experienced a heat stroke should not return to sporting activity for at least a week, or two.

Death rates have been as high as 80 per cent in the past, but are more likely to be around 15 per cent if the condition is immediately and effectively taken care of. Without immediate treatment, seizures, kidney failure, heart damage, breathing problems, a reduction in the effectiveness of the immune system, and of course, death, can result.

What to Do About Heat-Related Problems
1. Recognize the temperature and humidity and take the required measures to reduce injury.

2. Drink a great deal of water and some fluid replacement drinks during the practice. There is no need to take salt tablets. Drink more than you think you need.
3. Wear cool clothing that allows perspiration to escape. White clothes will deflect the sun better.
4. Exercise during the cooler part of the day; morning is better.

COLD-RELATED PROBLEMS

Drying-Out of the Mucous Membranes

One of the problems of exercising in cold air is that it may dry out the mucous membranes, because cold air cannot hold as much water vapour as warmer air. Wearing a mask that traps the exhaled water vapour and can re-humidify the inhaled air can reduce this problem.

Frostnip

Most cold-related problems have to do with the effect of the cold on the skin.

Frostnip occurs when the ends of the fingers, toes, ears or nose are chilled. The skin is very cold and somewhat stiffened. Warm the affected area slowly. This is best done using your hands. The armpits may be used to warm chilled fingers.

Frostbite

Frostbite can begin at temperatures as high as 31 degrees Fahrenheit (–0.5 degrees centigrade). The most likely victims are people who have previously had the problem, for whom the rate is doubled. Frostbite can be superficial, or deep and severe.

When frostbite has occurred, gently warm the area. Do not rub it to increase circulation, because the rubbing can destroy the cells which have been frozen. A warm bath (104 to 108 degrees Fahrenheit, 40-42 degrees centigrade) will help. For severe frostbite, the victim should be hospitalized where the re-warming can be done under proper supervision.

Proper protection is essential to avoid the problem and is doubly important to those who have already had one case of frostbite. Wear layers of wool clothing, vapour barrier clothing, adequate gloves or mittens, and a face mask, if necessary. Outdoor practice and games are not recommended if the ambient temperature is –4 degrees Fahrenheit (–20 degrees centigrade), or if the wind chill factor is too great.

Hypothermia

Hypothermia is a generalized body cooling. While the cooling is not as dangerous to body tissues as heat, there is still a danger of death. It can occur quickly, such as when a person falls into very cold water, or slowly, as when the person is exposed to low air temperatures for a length of time.

Dehydration often occurs, because the blood flow to the skin is reduced. This increases the volume of blood in the organs; the liver senses the increased blood volume, and removes the excess water from the blood, resulting in less total water in the body.

The people most susceptible to this type of problem are older athletes (because of their reduced metabolic activity), young athletes with large skin surfaces but less body mass (for example, tall, thin teenagers), hypoglycaemic or diabetic athletes, and those with reduced glycogen stores (energy

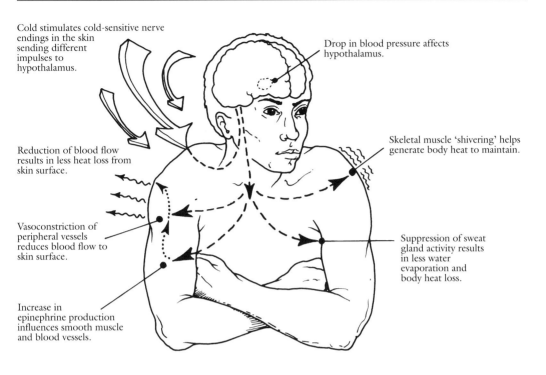

Cold stimulates cold-sensitive nerve endings in the skin sending different impulses to hypothalamus.

Drop in blood pressure affects hypothalamus.

Reduction of blood flow results in less heat loss from skin surface.

Skeletal muscle 'shivering' helps generate body heat to maintain.

Vasoconstriction of peripheral vessels reduces blood flow to skin surface.

Suppression of sweat gland activity results in less water evaporation and body heat loss.

Increase in epinephrine production influences smooth muscle and blood vessels.

Fig 98. Cold and the body.

reserves) due to physical exertion or shivering.

Hypothermia can begin in outside temperatures of less than 64 degrees Fahrenheit (18 degrees centigrade), especially if it is wet. Long-distance races and other endurance events in these low temperatures can cause problems. Those who take part in swimming, free diving, or SCUBA are particularly prone to hypothermia, because water conducts heat away from the body thirty-two times more rapidly than air does.

The symptoms, in addition to feeling cold and shivering, may include poor judgement, confusion, muscle stiffness and unconsciousness. If hypothermia is diagnosed, get the person to hospital as quickly as possible, where special internal and external warming methods can be used. Cold wet clothes should be removed, and the body insulated against further cold, in a warm room.

What to Wear in the Cold

Cold-related problems are best prevented by dressing in wool or polypropylene clothing. Cotton is not recommended, because it holds perspiration and increases the heat loss through conduction. The clothing should be

WIND SPEED MPH	WHAT IT EQUALS ON EXPOSED FLESH											
	50	40	30	20	10	0	−10	−20	−30	−40	−50	−60
	WHAT THE THERMOMETER READS (DEGREES F)											
40	26	10	−6	−21	−37	−53	−69	−85	−100	−116	−132	−148
35	27	11	−4	−20	−35	−49	−67	−82	−98	−113	−129	−145
30	28	13	−2	−18	−33	−48	−63	−79	−94	−109	−125	−140
25	30	16	0	−15	−29	−44	−59	−74	−88	−104	−118	−133
20	32	18	4	−10	−25	−39	−53	−67	−82	−96	−110	−121
15	36	22	9	−5	−18	−36	−45	−58	−72	−85	−99	−112
10	40	28	16	4	−9	−21	−33	−46	−58	−70	−83	−95
5	48	37	27	16	6	−5	−15	−26	−36	−47	−57	−68
CALM	50	40	30	20	10	0	−10	−20	−30	−40	−50	−60

Little danger if properly clothed	Danger of freezing exposed flesh	Great danger of freezing exposed flesh

Fig 99. The 'wind chill' factor.

Blueness or puffiness of the skin	Apathy
Drowsiness	Uncontrolled shivering
Vague, slow, slurred, thick speech	Poor judgement, dizziness, blackouts, unconsciousness
Apparant exhaustion	Frequent stumbling, lurching gait
Decreased heart and respiratory rate, weak and irregular pulse	Memory lapses, disorientation, mental confusion

Fig 100. Signs and symptoms of hypothermia.

in layers to reduce the body's heat loss, and the absorption of the cold from the outside. Layered clothing has better insulating qualities than a few thick articles of clothing. The multiple layers use the trapped air between the layers of the clothing for insulation. Effective gloves or mittens, a warm hat and/or ear muffs, wool socks, and a woollen or other type of mask are all important.

PROBLEMS AT ALTITUDE

Altitude Sickness

Altitude sickness comes about as a result of the reduced amount of oxygen in the atmosphere high above sea level. It is most common in altitudes above 7,000 feet (2,100 metres), but can occur at only 4,000 feet (1,200 metres). About 30 per cent of people will experience it when they go to 10,000 feet (3,000 metres), and 75 per cent will be similarly affected at altitudes over 15,000 feet (4,500 metres).

Increasing altitude by only 1,000 feet (300 metres) per day would probably not have a negative effect, but going directly to, say, a ski resort above 8,000 feet (2,400 metres) might cause difficulties.

Sleeping at an altitude of over 8,000 feet (2,400 metres) can also bring on the symptoms. In going to a high altitude, it is best to keep the increases in altitude, for sleeping purposes, to less than 1,500 feet per night (450 metres). 'Periodic breathing', in which the breathing pattern is not rhythmical during sleep, may develop at altitude. This disturbs the quality of sleep, and especially the deepest sleep. It is during this deepest sleep period (the 'delta' phase) that the most restful sleep occurs. It generally takes two to four days to adjust to altitudes around 8,000 feet 2,400 metres. It is generally believed

that the old adage of 'sleep low, train high' is a true one.

Flying, skiing, hang gliding, and any other activity at altitude – for example, the Olympic Games in Mexico City – can all cause an athlete problems related to the reduced oxygen pressure. The effects of the lack of oxygen generally occur within eight to twenty-four hours. The symptoms for moderate altitude sickness include headaches (especially in the front of the head), insomnia, nausea, and breathing problems. More severe symptoms can include reduced food intake, vomiting, tiredness, and worse breathing problems, even at rest.

The most common treatments include drinking more fluids (water, not alcohol), analgesics such as aspirin, higher carbohydrate intake, rest, and, if not yet at the final altitude, a slower ascent to that final altitude.

High-Altitude Pulmonary Oedema

High-altitude pulmonary oedema is a more serious problem than altitude sickness. While it can occur as low as 8,000 feet (2,400 metres), it is most likely at altitudes over 13,000 feet (4,000 metres). The symptoms include poor judgement, memory loss, hallucinations, reduced concentration, slowed reaction time, lack of co-ordination, disorientation, bleeding in the eyes, and possibly coma and death.

The victim must rest and be taken to an altitude below 6,500 feet (1,900 metres). If oxygen is available it should be given, and drugs (Diamox) may help. Often, bringing the victim only 1,000 feet (300 metres) lower will begin a rapid improvement, and a drop of 3,000 feet (900 metres) will almost certainly result in a great reduction of the symptoms.

If altitude sickness has occurred previously, it is important to be careful going up to the same altitude again. Often, a few days at 6,500 feet (1,900 metres) will ease the transition to a higher altitude. If an athlete must compete at the higher altitude, a doctor may decide to give medication, such as Nifedipine, to ease the transition prior to and during the increase in altitude.

AIR POLLUTION

Air pollution is most common in urban areas, especially near well-travelled roads (carbon monoxide, lead, oxides of nitrogen and sulphuric acid), indoor ice rinks (oxides of nitrogen), and swimming pools (chlorine forming chloroform). Oil refineries as well as cars emit carbon monoxide, sulphuric acid, carbon dioxide, oxides of nitrogen, and lead. Runners in urban areas generally have high levels of lead in their blood, while the levels of blood lead are being reduced in the general population because of the use of lead-free petrol.

Air

Air is a limited resource. Normal air contains 21 per cent oxygen. When the percentage of oxygen in the air drops to 16 per cent, the brain is affected. Life cannot be supported if the oxygen level drops to 6 per cent.

Air pollution is nothing new. In the thirteenth century, it was against the law to burn coal in London while Parliament was in session. Air pollution has occurred from natural causes such as volcanoes, methane from swamps, dumps, and mining, and man-made causes have included toxic gases of carbon monoxide from the smoke of any kind of fire. Factories often emit chlorine gas and hydrocarbons. The phenomenon is not limited to urban areas; in primitive New Guinea, it has been found that in the huts of the villages there is a high concentration of air pollution, because of the fires built in the huts.

Motor vehicles burn more than 600 million gallons of gasoline each day in the US. This burning increases nearly all the pollutants in the air. In a city such as Los Angeles, automobiles and trucks produce 45 tons of aerosols, 585 tons of nitrogen oxide, 35 tons of sulphur dioxide, and 9,775 tons of carbon monoxide daily. Aircraft add an additional 19 tons of nitrogen oxide and 190 tons of carbon monoxide to that city's air.

Sulphur Compounds

Sulphur dioxide plus oxygen in the air becomes sulphur trioxide, which is more irritating than sulphur dioxide. The sulphur trioxide then combines with water vapour in the air to become sulphuric acid. (The chemical formula is $2SO_2 + O_2 = 2SO_3 + 2H_2O/2 H2SO_4$.) Coal, which is 1 to 5 per cent sulphur, is a major contributor to the sulphur dioxide content of the air. Sulphuric acid is very destructive to lung tissue. The sulphuric acid is also picked up through convection and becomes an ingredient in acid rain, which has become a problem in northern latitudes.

Carbon Monoxide

Carbon monoxide is released by burning anything. In cities it is primarily the burning of petrol or gasoline which is the major problem. The carbon monoxide (CO) is picked up by the haemoglobin in the blood. (Haemoglobin is the iron-based compound in the red blood cells which carries the oxygen from the lungs to the tissues.) The haemoglobin is then rendered useless in transporting necessary oxygen to the tissues. The heart must work harder and the blood pressure is increased, which increases strain on the heart.

Carbon monoxide in the blood is increased while driving a car, standing on a busy road, or just living in the city. In downtown Los Angeles, carbon monoxide has been measured as high as 400 parts per million. At 600 parts per million, drowsiness occurs, and at 1,000 parts per million, a person could go into a coma. Exposure to 1 per cent carbon monoxide in the air for five minutes could be fatal.

Among the symptoms of carbon monoxide poisoning (high carbo-oxi-haemoglobin levels) are: headache, nausea, dizziness, and a lack of muscular co-ordination. They are most likely to occur in people who work near cars – mechanics, policemen, and car-park attendants. They can certainly also have a serious effect on athletes training in polluted air, who are breathing in much more air per hour than average.

Ozone

Ozone is a type of molecule of oxygen which performs the function of filtering out some of the harmful radiation of the sun. This occurs in the upper atmosphere 8 to 30 miles (13-45km) above the earth's surface. Since the mid-1980s, there has been a 5 per cent loss of ozone in the stratosphere due to the use of chlorofluo-rocarbons (CFCs) from spray cans, and the freon used in air-conditioning gases. This increases the amount of ultraviolet (UV) light which reaches the ground, causing faster skin ageing and serious skin cancer, and cataracts, the hardening of the lens in the eye. The reduction of the ozone layer makes it even more important for athletes exercising outdoors to use an effective sun block, and wear a hat.

Not all ozone is found high in the upper atmosphere. At the lower elevations, ozone is an irritating element of smog. It breaks down some membranes in plants, causing them to lose water and nutrients. Unable to repair themselves, the plants then die. This happens when the concentration of ozone is one to five parts per 10 million parts of air. Rats exposed to ozone develop lesions in their bronchial tubes and lungs, but do not seem to develop cancer (Boorman, G.A. *et al.*, 'Toxicology and carcinogenesis studies of ozone', Toxicology and Pathology, 22:5, September 1994, pp. 545–554). Ozone probably also has negative effects on humans.

Various studies have indicated that some people may be able to build a tolerance to the negative effects of ozone. Residents of Los Angeles seem to have developed some capacities for rebuilding lung tissues damaged by the pollutant. People with chronic emphysema, respiratory diseases, or those who have not been exposed to smog (such as many residents of Canada), do not have this capacity.

Lead

Approximately three million tons of lead have been released into the atmosphere since it was added to petrol or gasoline in 1923. Poisoning begins when the level of lead in the body reaches 0.8 parts per million. Recent samples have shown that the average person in the US has between 0.05 and 0.4 parts per million in the blood. The blood concentration is generally higher in areas near large numbers of cars. So far, no known deaths have occurred due to airborne lead poisoning.

Smog

Smog (a term coined from the words smoke and fog) is visible evidence of the extent of air pollution. In 1952, there was a smog in London so thick that people could not see their hands in front of their faces. The sulphur dioxide content reached 5-10 per cent, killing many people. People left their cars in the middle of the street; they slept in doorways because they didn't know how to get home; several people drowned in the River Thames, tripping over the unseen guard rail. In Donora, Pennsylvania, some years ago, a deadly smog increased the death rate by 2,000 per cent.

Smog is caused by stagnant air becoming polluted, primarily by car exhausts. These stagnant air masses can be caused by high-pressure areas which stop the flow of air. They can be normal weather fronts or they can occur as layers of hot air holding the cooler but dirtier air near ground level. When the latter occurs, it is called a temperature inversion layer.

The Temperature Inversion Layer

The temperature inversion layer increases the effects of air pollution. Normally air gets cooler at each higher level of altitude (approximately three degrees Fahrenheit for each thousand feet). At some times or some places, a warm layer of air forms over the cooler air and holds the dirty air closer to the ground. These inversion layers may form at an altitude of a few hundred feet to a few thousand feet. This is the type of phenomenon which increases the intensity of smog in London and Los Angeles.

Both cities have done a great deal to reduce air pollution. London converted most fireplaces from coal to other fuels. They don't have their famous smogs as often now. Los Angeles has required tough auto and industry standards to reduce air pollutants. In spite of more people moving there in the last 20 years, air pollution is reduced.

Effects of Air Pollution

Lung cancer and emphysema are the most common effects of air pollution; but increased carbon monoxide levels could certainly increase heart attack rates by increasing blood pressure and making the cardiovascular system less effective. People living in urban areas have twice the lung cancer rate of those who live in rural areas.

Sulphuric acid has been found to be a constrictor of the bronchial tubes leading to the lungs. This is a particular problem for those with asthma, but also affects many other people. With the bronchial tubes reduced in diameter, it is more difficult to inhale and the necessary oxygen is decreased – thereby cutting endurance.

The oxides of nitrogen also reduce the ability of the respiratory organs (bronchial tubes and lungs) to function effectively. They also increase the risk of infection.

Nitrogen is increased where propane (liquid nitrogen) is used as a fuel, such as in indoor ice rinks where the machines which clear and smooth the ice are generally propane-powered.

Reducing your workout risk can be done with intelligent planning. Meteorological reports give the air pollution level for the next day. When it is high, workouts should be reduced or eliminated. Training is safer if done away from heavy traffic, and before or after rush hour.

CHAPTER 14
Degenerative Diseases

THE BENEFITS AND RISKS OF SPORT

Most people in developed countries die of 'chronic' or 'degenerative' diseases, rather than communicable, or infectious ones. The top killers are diseases of the heart, cancer, stroke, respiratory problems (bronchitis, emphysema, and asthma), and diabetes.

In many cases, our lifestyle can contribute to the development of the disease. We eat too much and/or exercise too little. Understanding more about how such diseases develop makes it possible to increase our chances of leading a longer healthier life by changing our habits.

Being involved in sports helps, but it can hurt, too. Aerobic sports (such as running, walking, swimming, cycling, rowing, and aerobics) make the most important contribution to a longer life, according to the most recent large-scale research. Not smoking cigarettes is second on the list. Team sports such as soccer, rugby, field hockey, lacrosse, basketball, and team handball can also help to prolong life. Not all sports contribute to longevity. American football, baseball, cricket and weight-lifting do not have a high aerobic component – but it is certainly better to participate in them than to watch sports on television!

Aerobic sports help longevity by reducing blood levels of certain blood fats (triglycerides and LDL cholesterol), increasing levels of the beneficial cholesterol-scavenging fat high-density lipoprotein (HDL), controlling diabetes and high blood pressure, reducing depression, and, for some, making stronger bones. Endurance exercise may also help to control body weight, and make the immune system more effective.

Although the overall benefits of exercise greatly outweigh any risk of harm from sport, it is true that sport can damage life sometimes. It can, for example, cause injury that can lead to permanent disability, for example, or it can put the participant more at risk from skin cancers, if he or she is frequently exercising outdoors, without proper sun protection. The risk of sudden death (normally from a heart attack) is increased during very strenuous activity such as squash.

Some 'dangerous' sports clearly increase the participant's chance of premature death. In recent years, two former graduate students of the Norwegian University of Sport and Physical Education have died in the pursuit of their sport. In 1995, a student who had written his master's thesis on parachuting died in a parachute jump. In March 1997, a student who had written his thesis on avalanches died in an avalanche while mountain climbing. That challenging aspect of the sport – the danger – may have been precisely the attraction for those participants. Statistically, the vast majority of sports pose no greater risk to the participant than riding in a car.

MEDICAL EXAMINATIONS

Pre-participation medicals rarely detect new problems in fit young people, but there is a good argument for using a screening questionnaire, and a simple physical check. The questionnaire asks about any incidence of sudden death (from heart attack) in a close family member before the age of fifty, and about collapse, sudden shortness of breath or palpitations during exercise. Medical conditions such as diabetes, high blood pressure, and chest diseases should be assessed, and can be screened for with a urine test and simple examination. An electrocardiogram (ECG) or chest x-ray may be needed for some sports such as scuba diving.

It is significant that the father of the well-known runner and author, Jim Fixx, died early of heart disease. Fixx thought that running was a 'cure-all', but a physical examination might have saved him from his early death.

CARDIO-VASCULAR PROBLEMS

The causes of heart attack and many cases of stroke are similar because in both cases the blood flow to the organ is slowed or stopped. This lack of blood results in the lack of oxygen and nutrients, so part of the heart muscle or brain tissue dies.

Heart Attack

Heart attack *(myocardial infarction)* occurs when one or more of the coronary arteries that bring blood to the heart muscle is blocked. Without that blood, the heart muscle will not have the oxygen that it needs, and will die. The muscle dies in the area forward of the blockage. The area damaged during a heart attack can be so small that the individual doesn't even know that a heart attack has occurred, or it can be so massive that the individual dies immediately.

Hardened Arteries

Hardened arteries *(atherosclerosis)* are a major contributor to both heart disease and stroke. When the inner layer of the artery hardens and thickens due to fatty deposits (plaques), it is called atherosclerosis. This is the hardening that is the most significant cause of heart attack and stroke.

High Blood Pressure

High blood pressure *(hypertension)* goes hand in hand with hardened arteries as a significant contributor to both heart disease and stroke. Hypertension can lead to heart attack, stroke, and kidney disease. Hypertension is of concern because of the harm it can do to the heart, kidneys, brain, and blood vessels, if it remains uncontrolled for long periods of time. The heart is the organ most commonly damaged by high blood pressure. The increased force required during each beat makes the heart muscle thicken and become abnormally enlarged. It also speeds the hardening of the arteries of the heart.

High blood pressure occurs when the blood vessels in the body are constricted, either by contraction of the muscles in the artery wall or a build-up of plaque in the arteries. The heart is then required to beat more forcefully than normal. This forceful beat increases the pressure of the blood flowing from the heart. Exercise can reduce the resting blood pressure, by reducing both plaque formation and artery wall muscle contraction.

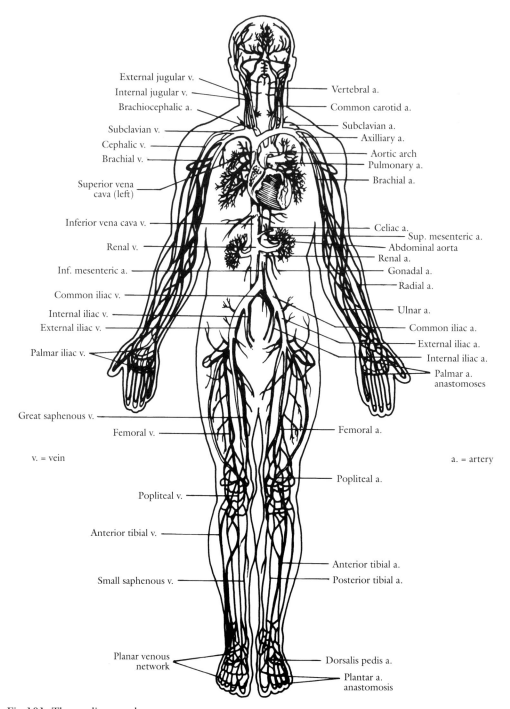

External jugular v.
Internal jugular v.
Brachiocephalic a.
Subclavian v.
Cephalic v.
Brachial v.
Superior vena cava (left)
Inferior vena cava v.
Renal v.
Inf. mesenteric a.
Common iliac v.
Internal iliac v.
External iliac v.
Palmar iliac v.

Vertebral a.
Common carotid a.
Subclavian a.
Axilliary a.
Aortic arch
Pulmonary a.
Brachial a.
Celiac a.
Sup. mesenteric a.
Abdominal aorta
Renal a.
Gonadal a.
Radial a.
Ulnar a.
Common iliac a.
External iliac a.
Internal iliac a.
Palmar a. anastomoses

Great saphenous v.
Femoral v.

v. = vein

Femoral a.

a. = artery

Popliteal v.

Popliteal a.

Anterior tibial v.

Small saphenous v.

Anterior tibial a.
Posterior tibial a.

Planar venous network

Dorsalis pedis a.
Plantar a. anastomosis

Fig 101. The cardio-vascular system.

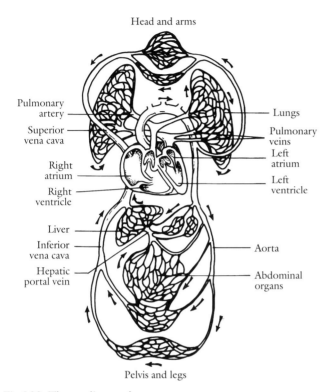

Fig 102. The cardiovascular system.

Blood pressure is easily checked, either with an automatic sphygmomanometer, which can be bought at most chemists, or routinely by a family doctor or practice nurse. A pressure of 110/70 is ideal and normal for many women, while 120/80 is generally considered to be normal and is common for many men; 140/90 is borderline high. Regular exercise, normal body weight, and reducing salt (sodium chloride) in the diet can all bring the blood pressure down naturally, but most doctors will treat blood pressure levels with drugs if it is consistently above 160/95. Generally, the lower the blood pressure the better – unless it gets so low that light-headedness is experienced. This may happen when it reaches 90/60 or lower.

Blood pressure may vary greatly during any one day, so a high reading is not conclusive. If it remains high, however, it may be dangerous, and a doctor should be consulted. Having an automatic meter at home makes it easy to get an accurate picture of your blood pressure.

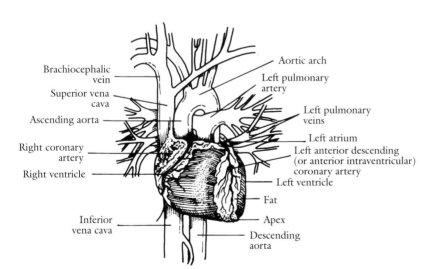

Fig 103. Major arteries and veins of the heart.

THE CAUSES OF VASCULAR PROBLEMS

The risk factors implicated in the development of both atherosclerosis and hypertension are the same. It is likely that one causes the other. Their possible causes include the following.

Heredity

Heredity is often responsible for the tendency to high blood pressure, and being overweight. In studies comparing children of both natural and adoptive parents, the parents with abnormal body weight or blood pressure gave birth to children who manifested the same symptoms. Adopted children in the same household tended to have normal readings, despite identical diets.

Inherited racial characteristics may also play a part. Among blacks, one in four have hypertension; interestingly, only one in 500 have the much-publicized sickle cell anaemia. Among whites, one person in eight is hypertensive. Even black children are found to have significantly higher blood pressure than white children do. The rise in black children's blood pressure often shows up as early as five years of age. Whether inherited or environmentally induced, blood pressure seems to be determined, to a large degree, early in life.

Environment

Particular types of environment and lifestyle are major causes of cardio-vascular disease. Being overweight, eating certain types of food, reactions to stress, cigarette smoking, and inadequate exercise are all possible contributors to cardio-vascular diseases.

Exercise that requires the heart to work hard for a reasonably long period of time is a positive factor in keeping the circulatory system functioning efficiently. There are various theories as to why it works, but the results of effective exercise are well established. Exercise aids in reducing the effects of stress, lowers harmful blood fats while raising the protective blood fats, and may increase the number of open blood vessels in the heart. These combined effects not only lessen the possibility of a heart attack, they also increase the chances of survival should a heart attack occur.

Smoking

Smoking has many negative effects on the circulatory system. Smokers have raised blood pressure and blood fats, and the carbon monoxide in their blood makes the blood less efficient. This makes the heart work much harder to circulate the required oxygen to the body. Smoking is directly responsible for between 100,000 and 200,000 heart attack deaths each year in the United States.

It is possible to reverse the effects of smoking on the circulator system. Five to ten years after giving up smoking, the ex-smoker's risk of heart disease is the same as that of someone who has never smoked.

When smoking is stopped, the blood pressure will generally fall, the amount of oxygen in each unit of blood will be increased, the artery hardening process will slow, and the amount of cholesterol in the blood will be reduced.

Being Overweight

Excess body fat increases the work of the heart. Every pound (0.5kg) of fat adds about 200 miles (300km) of capillaries that must be filled with blood so that the fat can be nourished. Being overweight increases the risk of high blood pressure, high blood cholesterol, and diabetes. The Body Mass Index (BMI) – the weight in kilograms divided by the height in metres squared – should be between 20–25. A very muscular athlete will be heavier, but a BMI of 25 to 30 in the average person suggests too much body fat, and a BMI above 30 indicates obesity, which is very dangerous to health.

Stress

Stress may be a factor in cardio-vascular diseases. It causes adrenalin secretion and high blood pressure, and an increase in stickiness of blood platelets, and all of these are known risk factors for heart problems. In one study, highly stressed men 'out-died' their low-stress counterparts by a 3 to 1 ratio over a five-year period.

Dr Hans Selye, director of the Institute of Experimental Medicine and Surgery at the University of Montreal, and perhaps the world's authority on stress, said, 'It is not the stress that is the problem, but how one reacts to stress. The trick is not to avoid stress, but to enjoy and master it.'

Diet

The subject of diet has been studied at great length. The positive effects of low-fat diets, and of diets low in sodium and high in potassium, are well known, but the addition of anti-oxidants is now also being recognized as an important step in reducing both heart disease and many cancers. Vitamins C and E and beta carotene, which is converted into vitamin A, as well as the mineral selenium, all have anti-oxidant properties. They are thought to reduce the damage in the artery walls that may precede the development of the atherosclerotic plaques in the arteries. (*See* Chapters 19 and 20.)

Fats in the Blood

Fats in the blood are considered to contribute significantly to hardened arteries. The most frequently studied blood fats are the lipoproteins, cholesterols, and the triglycerides.

The major types of lipoproteins are:
1. heavy-density lipoproteins (HDL) which transport cholesterol from the body's tissues to the liver, where it can be eliminated;
2. low-density lipoproteins (LDL) which take cholesterol from the liver to the tissues; they contain few triglycerides; 60 to 80 per cent of the body's cholesterol is carried by the LDL;
3. very low-density lipoproteins (VLDL), which contain primarily triglycerides, with a little cholesterol. They carry triglycerides to the tissues and fat of the body, where they can be used for energy.

Cholesterol is a waxy substance used in many of the body's chemical processes. It is required in everyone in certain amounts. When there is too much cholesterol being carried by the LDLs, some can be deposited in the artery walls. This is the build-up which we call atherosclerosis (artery 'fat scarring', or hardened arteries). Seventy to eighty per cent of cholesterol is made in the body, primarily by the liver, from saturated fats that are eaten; the remaining 20 to 30 per cent of the blood's cholesterol is eaten in the form of cholesterol in animal products.

The HDLs (the 'good' lipoproteins) are associated with lower cardio-vascular risk because they are able to get rid of the cholesterols that, if allowed to stay in the blood, can develop plaques in the arteries of the heart, neck and brain. Women tend to have more HDL than men, because of the oestrogen they produce. Oestrogen replacement after menopause can continue this protection, otherwise a woman's heart attack risk will rise as she grows older.

The LDLs (the 'bad' lipoproteins) carry cholesterol to the tissues. Some of this may be implanted in the arteries, hardening and narrowing them. This process seems to need oxygenation in order to occur, the free oxygen radicals change the fat in the LDL. Once it is changed, it can be deposited into the artery walls. Both HDL and the anti-oxidant vitamins (A, C and E) reduce the rate of this oxygenation.

Triglycerides are the most common type of blood fat. While they are found in some foods, such as luncheon meats and shellfish, they are generally constructed in the liver from carbohydrates, such as sugars, in the diet. Much more is known about cholesterol in the blood, but some experts think that the triglycerides may be even more harmful.

ASPIRIN

Aspirin reduces the risk or heart disease by making the blood less likely to clot. It also reduces inflammation, which some people now believe is a major cause of the fat build-up in the arteries.

CANCERS

The risk of some cancers can be increased due to the environmental effects of exercise; the biggest risk is skin cancer. Remember that anti-oxidant vitamins can increase the effectiveness of the immune system and thereby reduce the effects of carcinogenic agents. Remember also that the value of

exercise in terms of general health far outweighs any risk.

Skin cancer is becoming more prevalent as the ozone layer is depleted by CFCs and other air pollutants, and as more recreational hours are spent in the sun. The worst skin damage occurs to those under 18, and serious cancers later in life are clearly related to severe sunburns early in life. It is particularly important, therefore, to protect young people from the harmful effects of the sun. A sun block with a protection factor (SPF) of at least 15 should be used. Make sure that it can block both the UV-A and the UV-B rays. Avoid going into the sun when it is at its highest point. Sunbeds are not recommended – the ultra-violet A (UV-A) rays of sunlamps and the sun can cause cancers in the same way as the more dangerous ultra-violet B (UV-B) radiation from the sun (which has always been the major concern).

While most skin cancers are benign and easily removed, there is a deadly type, called melanoma. If it is localized on the skin, the five-year survival rate is 90 per cent, but that survival rate drops to 55 per cent if the cancer has spread to nearby organs, and to 14 per cent if it has spread to more distant organs.

The outer layer of skin, the epidermis, is made up of several types of cells that can be affected by the ultra-violet rays of the sun. Basal cell carcinoma (which sometimes metastasizes) is the most common type of skin cancer, affecting 500,000 people each year. Squamous cell carcinoma also affects hundreds of thousands. It is caused not only by the sun's rays but also by hydrocarbons found in some oils, tars, and asphalts.

Some serious skin cancers, or melanomas, appear as darker spots on the skin. The more serious are quite dark, like moles, and are likely to have a rougher texture. There are different types, as follows:

1. Caucasians, particularly women, are likely to develop a melanoma from a normal mole, which becomes irregular in both shape and size; this type accounts for 70 per cent of all cases;
2. brown-black, blue-black, or dark brown lesions are more common among Asians and Africans, and are likely to occur on the hands, feet, or mucous membranes;
3. women over 50 who have spent years in the sun suffer from a third type;
4. lesions looking like blood blisters, in colours ranging from nearly white to blue-black are more common among men, and start under the skin.

A monthly self-examination, preferably done with a friend, is the best way to spot an early cancer. Starting from the scalp, check for dark spots on all parts of the body – under the hair, on the face and neck, in the mouth, behind the ears, on the genitals. A common place for such cancers to start in women is on the lower legs.

ALLERGIES

Allergies affect millions of people, who sneeze from pollen in the summer, wheeze from asthma, or itch, swell, or develop hives from any number of substances that they breathe, eat, touch, or even receive by injection. Allergens are the culprits, and they affect different people is different ways. Milk is an allergen to some people.

People who exhibit allergies usually have very high levels of an antibody called immunoglobulin E, or IgE. When IgE antibodies meet with mast cells in the body, they release histamines and other chemicals that cause the smooth muscles to contract and blood vessels to dilate. The tissues surrounding the blood vessels then swell. If this hap-pens in the nose, it results in hay fever; if in the bronchial tubes leading to the lungs, a type of asthma. A bee sting can trigger such a massive histamine reaction that the victim can suffocate. In fact, bee stings cause more deaths each year in the United States than do rattlesnake bites.

If you suffer allergic reactions, a doctor or an allergist can study your health history and give you tests that may help in deciding what is affecting you. Eliminating the culprits from your surroundings can decrease the number of allergic attacks. If you are allergic to feathers, switch to synthetic-filled pillows; if you are found to be allergic to a certain antibiotic, don't take that medication; if you are allergic to substances outdoors, keep your doors closed and buy an air filtration system.

Hay fever (*allergic rhinitis*) is the most common allergy. Sufferers are allergic to airborne particles (pollens, moulds, or spores) or possibly the household dust, animal dandruff, musty books, or furniture. It is uncomfortable, and can affect athletic performance.

Asthma affects millions of people and causes many deaths each year. The breathing difficulties, due primarily to muscle spasms in the bronchial tubes, are the effect of the allergens upon the asthmatic person. The same types of allergens that may start hay fever can spark an asthmatic attack in some people, as can such foods as milk, eggs, seafood, nuts, and chocolate. Exercise can also bring on the symptoms of asthma. Exercise-induced asthma, a spasm of the bronchial tubes (*bronchospasm*), occurs in 90 per cent of asthmatics, 40 per cent of people with nose allergies and 15 per cent of people without either of these conditions. It is more common among those who are overweight. It occurs most often when people exercise strenuously in cold, dry air. Just four or five minutes of soccer or distance running can bring on the symptoms. When the air is warmer and moist, it is less likely to happen, and swimming is therefore generally better tolerated.

Anti-histamines may often give relief from allergic reactions, as they counteract the hist-amines and relieve the symptoms. For the recreational athlete, anti-histamines that do not cause drowsiness are often effective. The International Olympic Committee has banned many drugs, including the decon-gestants that can temporarily reduce the symptoms of exercise-induced bronchial problems (but are not a good long-term treatment). Olympic athletes need to be under the care of a doctor who is aware of the IOC rules.

ARTHRITIS

Arthritis (an inflammation of the joints) affects millions of people. Half of the popu-lation over 65 suffers from some type of arthritis, of which there are about one hun-

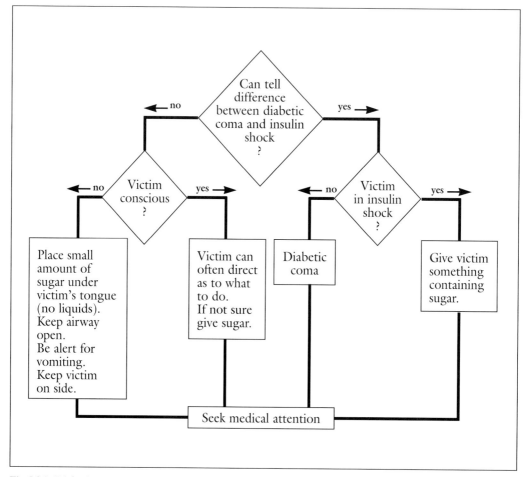

Fig 104. Diabetic emergencies.

dred types. The major categories of the disease are traumatic arthritis and osteoarthritis.

Traumatic arthritis is due to injury, including sports injuries, to the joints. Knees damaged in football or basketball are an example. Car accidents can cause whiplash, which can result in an arthritic condition in the neck. Osteoarthritis is wear and tear of the joints. It is the most common type of arthritis, affecting millions of people, usually those over 50 years of age. There is a strong hereditary link. Joint replacement, particularly of the hips and knees, is needed in severe cases. Moderate, low-impact exercise, such as walking, swimming, or cycling, has been shown to reduce symptoms, while increasing fitness.

Diabetes

Diabetes affects the pancreas, causing a deficiency of insulin, which metabolizes sugar. The symptoms of diabetes include excess thirst, increased output of urine, increased weight loss, and fatigue.

There are two general types of diabetes. Type I, or *insulin-dependent diabetes mellitus* (IDDM), previously called 'juvenile onset diabetes', occurs when the body is not able to manufacture insulin to metabolize the blood sugar. Type II, or *non-insulin dependent diabetes mellitus* (NIDDM), formerly called 'maturity onset diabetes', occurs when the amount of insulin produced is insufficient, or the cells become resistant to using it. This type is more likely to develop after the age of 40.

About 10 per cent of diabetics have Type I diabetes, which, while more common in the young, can occur in very old people. Type II often happens in overweight people, and even in overweight children; it can be controlled by diet and possibly by giving insulin. Although Type II is more likely to start in older people, it can occur in the young.

Diabetes is hereditary (it is estimated that about 45 million people carry the genetic capability of transmitting the disease), but it can be brought on more rapidly by environmental factors. Many people have the disease without knowing it. Since diet and exercise play a big part in Type II diabetes, people who live healthily may not develop any symptoms. In a study among 20,000 physicians, it was found that exercising once a week reduced the incidence of diabetes by 28 per cent, while exercising two to four times a week reduced it by 38 per cent (*Journal of American Medical Assn.*, Vol. 268 (1) July 1, 1992). About 75 per cent of people with Type II diabetes are obese, that is, at least 20 per cent overweight.

Osteoporosis

Osteoporosis (brittle bones) is a condition most often found in post-menopausal women, particularly those with smaller bones. Due to a lack of oestrogen (because of menopause), a lack of calcium in the diet, and a lack of weight-bearing activities such as weight lifting or walking, the bones begin to lose their structure. In some people, this shows as an extreme curvature of the upper back, due to the loss of bone in the vertebrae in the neck and thoracic areas. This forces the head downwards. More commonly it is seen in the thinning of the upper part of the thigh bone. Most broken hips of older people are caused by this bone loss.

Bones are active tissues, giving off and replacing calcium continually. At about the age of 35, women's bones begin to become less dense; the same thing happens a little later in men. After menopause, women's bone loss is increased because of the lack of oestrogen. By age 65 the average woman has lost 26 per cent of her bone density, while the average man has lost 9 per cent. The best methods of reducing the risk are:

1. a lifelong high intake of calcium (preferably non-fat milk or cheese), and/or calcium supplements. While the normal RDA for calcium is 800mg, many experts suggest that post-menopausal women should take 1,500mg daily (*University of California Wellness Letter*, July 1993, pp. 4–5);
2. weight-bearing exercise such as dancing, gardening, housework, walking and running; (yoga and swimming do not qualify);
3. not smoking;
4. drinking alcohol only in moderation;
5. considering hormone replacement therapy after the menopause;

Heredity plays a part in the potential for developing the condition. Small-boned people, particularly Asians and Caucasians, are at risk. Black women seem to have higher bone density, and are less at risk.

Varicose Veins

Varicose veins affect many people, particularly women. The valves that prevent the blood from moving downwards start to leak. This means the pumping action of the calf muscle is inefficient at moving blood back up the veins, which bulge and become tortuous.

Varicose veins may occur in people who are very muscular, and in pregnant women – the pressure of the uterus makes it more difficult for the blood to pass through the abdominal area, creating additional pressure on the valves of the veins. In many cases, the tendency towards varicose veins due to weak or malformed valves is inherited. Environmental factors can also contribute to varicose veins. People who are overweight or do heavy lifting will often have varicose veins.

To reduce the severity of varicose veins, it is best to exercise, walk, or swim, but not to stand or sit for too long. Good muscle activity will help to massage the blood back through the veins and towards the heart. Elevating the feet, above the level of the chest, uses gravity to assist the blood in its flow towards the heart. If the varicose veins are very large, it is possible for doctors to operate or use injections to shrink the veins.

CHAPTER 15

Infectious Diseases

Infectious or communicable diseases can be 'caught' from another living being, human or animal. In the developed world, infectious diseases do not kill in the way that they do in undeveloped countries. Vaccines and antibiotics have reduced or eliminated the chances of deformity and death from many of these diseases. In the eighteenth century, smallpox caused 10 per cent of all deaths, and every five or ten years it became an epidemic. It killed its victims, marked them with scars, or left them deaf or blind. The discovery of a vaccine enabled elimination of the disease.

Obviously, it is important for athletes and sportspeople to steer clear of any diseases that can reduce workout time and perhaps take them away from competition.

INFECTION

Infectious or communicable diseases are caused by *pathogens* (mainly *viruses, bacteria, fungi* and small *parasites*). These may be transmitted by touch, through the air in an *aerosol* (like the common cold), by eating infected foods or drinking contaminated water (traveller's diarrhoea), or by a bite (rabies and malaria). For a communicable disease to be passed on, the situation must be as follows:

- there must be a number of *pathogens* (germs or larger biological organisms);

- they must be in sufficient numbers to be able to infect a *reservoir;*
- they must be able to be removed from that reservoir by a *vector* (the method by which the pathogen is transmitted);
- they must be removed to the port of entry of a new organism, which is then infected.

For example, a sufficient number of respiratory infection-causing viruses in the nose of one person are carried out by a sneeze, on tiny airborne droplets of water (the *aerosol*), then breathed into the nose of another person, starting a new infection.

PATHOGENS

There are several types of disease-causing organisms, or pathogens.

Viruses

Viruses are smaller than cells, and can be seen only through an electron microscope. They are not capable of living alone so must reproduce and live within living cells. Viruses cause upper respiratory infections (colds), influenza, infectious mononucleosis, infectious hepatitis chickenpox, measles, HIV (Aids), viral pneumonia, warts, and cold sores (fever blisters). They are not killed by antibiotics.

119

Bacteria

Bacteria are one-celled, plant-like organisms that generally live between the cells of a host. Many are harmless or even useful (such as most of those living in the intestine), but others can produce extremely harmful poisons and destroy body cells. The major types of bacteria are cocci, which are spherical bacteria; they can act singly, in pairs *(diplococcus)*, in bunches or clusters *(staphylococcus)*, or in chains *(streptococcus)*. *Baccilli* are rod-shaped, *spirilli* are corkscrew-shaped. Bacteria cause such diseases as pneumonia, syphilis, gonorrhea, strep throat (streptococcal infections), toxic shock syndrome, boils (staphylococcal infections), Legionnaires' disease, tuberculosis, and Lyme disease.

Fungi

Fungi are primitive plants. They can be single-celled, like yeast, or have many cells, like moulds. They are like plants but do not contain chlorophyll. They are most commonly found on the skin, as in athlete's foot and other sorts of ringworm. They may also be found in the lungs. Fungal diseases include athlete's foot, ringworm, and the vaginal infection *candidiasis (monilia)*.

Protozoa

Protozoa are single-celled animals. Protozoan-caused diseases include malaria, the vaginal infection *trichomoniasis,* amoebic dysentery, African sleeping sickness, and several types of intestinal diseases. These are particularly common in South America, South-East Asia, and parts of central Africa.

Parasitic Worms

Parasitic worms, including tapeworms, roundworms or flukes, can also be disease-causing organisms. One disease caused by parasitic worms is *elephantiasis,* a not uncommon disease in some developing countries. Hookworm is a problem for one-quarter of the world's population, but is not prevalent in the western world. Threadworms are the most common parasitic disorder in some developed countries.

DEFENCES AGAINST COMMUNICABLE DISEASES

There are several defences against disease. On a communal level, this includes treating sewage, purifying water supplies, pasteurizing milk, inspecting meat, and developing vaccines.

The individual has several methods of self-protection from communicable diseases. For example, tears will be produced in the eye if a foreign body enters it; the skin and the mucous membranes prevent pathogens or germs from entering the body; the *cilia* of the respiratory tract prevent a good deal of dirt and micro-organisms from entering the lungs (90 per cent of inhaled microbes are expelled within an hour; the acid in the stomach helps to destroy many of the pathogens that are ingested; the body temperature increase, or an inflammation, may kill some of the germs, or dilute the toxins by increasing the blood flow.

If the disease does progress, white blood cells (such as *macrophages*) attack some of the invading pathogens, and this attack is more effective if other white cells *(lymphocytes)* have produced antibodies which attach to the pathogen. Other white cells *(T cells)* can kill body cells infected with viruses, especially if antibodies are attached. After the infection has been eradicated, some specially primed lymphoctes remain (in the glands or lymph nodes), so that if the same germ is encountered again, antibodies are produced very quickly and the germ is destroyed before it can get established. Immunization primes the white cells in a similar way, and there is evidence that exercise also stimulates the immune system in a more general way.

THE MOST PREVALENT DISEASES

The major disease problems in the world are malaria, tuberculosis, HIV, and cholera. These are all infectious, or communicable, diseases, which could be controlled but remain uncontrolled in many of the undeveloped nations. In the developed world, sexually transmitted diseases are a major infectious disease problem. There are many other infectious diseases, both serious and minor, which can be easily caught, and it is worth taking all precautions to avoid coming into contact with them.

The Common Cold

The common cold is the name given to upper respiratory tract infections, that is, infections in the nose and related organs. There are about 200 organisms, particularly viruses *(rhinoviruses)*, which cause the symptoms that we call a cold. As we all know, the most common symptoms are likely to be a runny nose, watery eyes, a slight fever, headache, general body aching, and sore throat.

Since a true cold is most likely to be caused by a virus, taking an antibiotic will not help. For viral infections, the body must fight the disease. Symptoms may be made less miserable by drinking more fluids, eating, and resting. Paracetamol or aspirin will reduce aches and fever. Cough syrups (which are depressants) and nasal decongestants (which are stimulants) will ease symptoms, but should not be used for more than a few days. Nasal decongestants will reduce the blood flow to the capillaries in the nose, so that breathing is easier; if they are used for more than four days, there is a rebound effect after stopping, with an increase in the amount of blood in those same capillaries and an increase in the nasal swelling. The stimulant decongestants (such as ephedrine) are banned in international athletes.

The 'above the neck and below the neck' rule is useful. If your symptoms are only above the neck (sore throat, runny nose, and swollen glands), the virus is localized to the lining of the nose and throat, and it is safe to do very light exercise. If the symptoms are below the neck (aching all over, fever, cough, and general malaise), then there is widespread infection and it is not safe to do any exercise at all. If exercise is done, the cold will take longer to get better, and there is an increased risk of *myocarditis* (viral infection of the heart).

It is wise to take as many precautions as possible to avoid catching a cold. It is often thought that sneezes and coughs transmit the disease, but it is more likely to be passed on through the hands. A recent study at the University of Virginia showed that only 8 per cent of people with colds expelled the virus through a cough or sneeze, but 40 per cent of sufferers had viruses on their hands, usually from blowing their noses or rubbing their eyes. A virus on the hands can be left on any surface and can be picked up by the next person who touches the surface, even after several hours. Handkerchiefs and paper tissues showed no signs of viruses three hours after being exposed to the viruses, but hard, dry surfaces were more apt to be transmitters. Try to avoid touching door knobs and bathroom hardware, and then touching your face. Wash hands frequently and avoid rubbing the eyes and picking the nose. Another precaution is to drink only out of your own cup or glass.

A cold cannot be caught from sitting in a draught, although this may contribute by cooling the body. In making the adjustment to the cold, the mucus on the mucous membranes may dry out, and this thinning of the mucus may allow germs already present to enter the body and begin the infection. Most people carry many of the viruses that can cause colds.

Not all upper respiratory symptoms are caused by colds. They are often caused by allergies, and an anti-histamine may reduce them. As previously mentioned, elite athletes should make sure they do not take drugs that are on the IOC banned list.

Sore Throat

Sore throats, or *pharyngitis,* affect many people. About 80 per cent of sore throats are caused by viral infections, or irritations from smoking, shouting, or coughing, and some are caused by bacteria.

One of the bacterial infections is a strep throat, which can be diagnosed only by having a throat culture sent to a laboratory. (This will take about 48 hours.) About 5 per cent of people are strep carriers. Although they may not have the strep infection, they may be able to transmit it to other people.

Among the indications of strep throat are accumulations of white or yellow mucus that may give a cobblestone appearance to the throat, lymph node enlargements under the jaw, a swelling and tenderness in the front of the neck, and a fever. Millions of people develop streptococcal infections and it is highly contagious, but easily cured with antibiotics. There is as yet no vaccine to stop these strep infections.

Influenza and Pneumonia

Influenza and pneumonia are major infections of the respiratory tract. Influenza is a virus-caused disease, so it cannot be treated by antibiotics. 'Flu' didn't become important until the late 1800s, and since then there have been periodic epidemics, sometimes killing as many as 40 million people, every two to four years. There are at least three different influenza viruses – Types A, B and C. Type A seems to cause the major epidemics – the Asian flu (1957), Hong Kong flu (1968), the A-Victorian flu, or the Swine flu. It is a communicable disease with which we should be concerned. The development of 'flus' from Asia has been associated with the combination of people, ducks, and pigs in the lifestyle of the rural Chinese; this seems to cause mutations of viruses, which cause many types of influenza.

Vaccines may be effective when given before exposure, and routine yearly immunization is recommended for people who have heart disease, lung ailments, diabetes, and for all people over 65. Many athletes have a yearly flu vaccination in order to reduce the chances of a major disruption to their training. Flu vaccines are effective in about 75 per cent of cases. Most of the deaths resulting from the flu are caused by complications from the disease, and not by the influenza viruses. Pneumonia is one of the major complications, although it can often be cured by antibiotics.

Pneumonia is on the increase. With flu, it is the fifth most significant cause of death. It is especially prevalent among children and people over 50. It can be caused either by bacteria (which can be cured by antibiotics), or by viruses (which cannot).

Pneumonia often begins three or four days after a cold, often with a sudden worsening of symptoms just as they were starting to improve. The symptoms include being cold with shaking chills, sweating, high fever, and chest pains. A pneumonia vaccine is now available.

Hepatitis

Hepatitis is a viral disease that attacks the liver. There are two main types of hepatitis – Type A, formerly called infectious hepatitis, and Type B, formerly called serum hepatitis. Only blood tests can distinguish the serum hepatitis from the infectious hepatitis. Recently, researchers have found other types of hepatitis which result in similar problems. Infectious hepatitis (Type A) is less serious than hepatitis B, but both are increasing in frequency, with many hundreds of thousands of cases annually.

Hepatitis A can be transmitted from faeces to mouth. Its most common sources are in sewage, polluted streams, rivers, and oceans. Swimmers in such waters may be infected. Oysters and other shellfish that have not been adequately cooked are often a source of the disease. Often, clams are served whole, including the guts. Each clam may contain as much as half a teaspoon of raw waste, which may contain human faecal material with bacteria and viral hepatitis. If

clams are steamed for about five minutes, it is possible to kill off the hepatitis virus. Hepatitis can also be spread from person to person in crowded living conditions, through contaminated air, food, or water.

Type B hepatitis has greatly increased recently through the contaminated needles of drug users. It can also happen when ears are pierced with inadequately sterilized instruments. Type B hepatitis is carried in any body fluid, such as blood, saliva, semen, or vaginal fluids, and it can be easily transmitted by sexual contact.

The symptoms of hepatitis are similar to those of flu, including fever, general weakness, loss of appetite, headache, and muscle pains. There may be orange urine or a lighter-coloured stool. Other symptoms include abdominal pain caused by a swelling of the liver and occasional vomiting and diarrhoea. These are usually followed by jaundice (a yellowing of the skin and/or the eyes).

The severity of the disease varies. Some people don't know they have it, for others it drags on for months, and some die. In a minority of cases, it leads to permanent damage of the liver such as cirrhosis and chronic hepatitis. There is some evidence that links hepatitis to increased risk of liver cancer. Hepatitis takes a long time to cure, but it is rarely fatal. The best cure seems to be plenty of rest, a balanced diet, and letting the disease run its course. People who have had the disease may still be carriers of it.

Glandular Fever

Glandular fever (infectious *mononucleosis*) is a viral disease that affects the white blood cells, caused by the Epstein-Barr virus. It is common in young people. Studies in the United States indicate a three- to four-fold increase in mononucleosis during the last five years. Most reported cases are in the 15 to 24 age group, but cases are increasing in other age groups.

The disease seems to be spread through personal contact such as kissing, and the common use of eating and drinking materials, because it can be transferred by the saliva. But fatigue and over exertion may also contribute to the illness. Symptoms may include any of the following: fever as high as 105 degrees Fahrenheit (40 degrees centigrade), chills, sore throat, abdominal pains, swollen lymph nodes, headache, stiff neck, tiredness, or a rash. Fatigue may last for many weeks or months.

Lyme Disease

Lyme Disease is caused by a bacterium of the spirochete variety. It is spread by infected ticks that live in the woods and on tall grasses. In some wooded areas, one person in six has become infected. If you run through the woods, or are involved in orienteering competitions, you may be exposed to these ticks.

It is not fatal but its effects can be serious, including arthritis, heartbeat irregularities (arrhythmia), severe headaches, and numbness. Early detection and treatment with antibiotics is important to reduce the chance of these severe symptoms developing.

Traveller's Diarrhoea

Traveller's diarrhoea (often referred to as 'Montezuma's Revenge', 'Delhi Belly' or the 'Haitian Hop', depending upon the country in which it is contracted) is often caused by a change in the intestinal flora when the traveller is not used to the local strain of *E. coli* bacteria. A sportsperson competing in other countries may want to take the following precautions to avoid this uncomfortable problem.

To prevent the disease:
1. minimize the dose of local bacteria taken by mouth; eat local foods sparingly at first, while building up a new intestinal environment;
2. eat well-cooked foods that have not been left standing after cooking; avoid rare meat, raw fish, and uncooked vegetables, especially lettuce;
3. always peel your own fruits; food handlers can easily contaminate uncooked foods;
4. avoid rich foods such as desserts, custards, potato salads, and milk products. Yogurt is the only universally safe milk product (except for pasteurized milk products), as harmful bacteria are killed in the curdling process;
5. drink only boiled or bottled liquids; avoid ice in your drinks (alcohol does not kill bacteria in water or ice cubes in a drink).

If you do get traveller's diarrhoea, make sure you drink plenty of fluids, ideally in the form of rehydration drinks. If the symptoms are severe, an antibiotic such as ciprofloxacin can shorten the duration of the illness.

Athlete's Foot

Athlete's foot, another common disease, is normally a fungus infestation that thrives in the moist area between the toes. Hot, sweaty or wet feet lead to a decrease in the acid on the surface of the skin, making it a perfect breeding ground for these fungi. Cracking, peeling or blistered skin between the toes may not be athlete's foot. It may be a reaction to shoe dye, chemicals in synthetic socks or stockings, or eczema.

Common shower rooms are a prime place to pick up athlete's foot. Wear rubber sandals or flip-flops when you shower. In order to prevent athlete's foot, don't wear tight or ill-fitting shoes. Non-porous socks or stockings should not be worn. Wide-open shoes and sandals allow the air to circulate around the feet, and cotton or wool socks help to absorb the moisture. If you wish to wear nylon or synthetic stockings, insert cotton between the toes, and dry your feet especially well after bathing. Using a medicated powder between the toes before a workout and after a shower can both prevent and cure athlete's foot.

CHAPTER 16

Psychology of Sports Participation

UNDERSTANDING STRESS

Everyone encounters stress. It may be life-threatening or a mere inconvenience. The manner in which it is handled can mean the difference between mental health and mental illness.

Stress can be said to be the response made by the mind and body when psychological requirements are too high (Don Frankl, paper delivered to the American Academy of Kinesiology, Washington, DC, April 1993). For example, reading a novel and reading a textbook in preparation for a test are both experiences in reading; but one may be stressful. Similarly, taking an exam and writing a letter, both experiences in writing, will cause different levels of stress. Stress can also be a physical condition; it could be caused by the effect of excess cold or heat on the body.

The cause of the stress is not the major concern, as much as the effect of that stress on the individual. An individual with a positive self-concept may be less likely to be overcome by a stressor, being more likely to feel in control, rather than have the stressor in control.

The Effects of Unhealthy Stress

The mind and body can react to stressors with anxiety, depression or hostility. These mental reactions can manifest themselves physically in diseases such as heart attack, high blood pressure, ulcers, neck and back pains, and asthma. Even cancers and other serious illnesses seem to be related to a lowering of the effectiveness of the immune system, a possible result of stress.

The recreational athlete is usually participating in sport for positive reasons – one of which may be to reduce the effects of stress at work. For the Olympic athlete, training and competition are equivalent to work, and the stress of high-level competition may be enormous. He or she must be specially trained and prepared to deal with that stress.

Good Stress and Bad Stress

Dr Hans Selye, the Canadian pioneer of stress research, tells us that there is good stress, or 'eustress', ('eu' from the Greek for 'good'), and bad stress, or 'distress'. We need stress in our lives, but we want to increase the eustress and decrease the distress. The excitement of playing a tennis match, or travelling to a new destination, and the stimulation of reading a good novel are eustresses. A long drive to work, hassles with people at home, a lack of challenge at work, boring sports practices, and continual injuries are distresses, which need to be eliminated or controlled.

Stress is natural for humans. Selye once observed that 'stress is the spice of life'. As we encounter stress, we must be able to cope with it, then, if possible, eliminate the negative stresses. Selye also captured the importance of stress in our lives when he wrote that 'man's ultimate aim in life is to express himself as fully as possible, according to his own lights, and to achieve a sense of security. To accomplish this, you must first find your optimal stress level, and then use your adaptation energy at a rate and in a direction adjusted to your innate qualifications and preferences.' (Selye, ibid. p. 110.)

Stresses may be handled by adapting to them, by eliminating them through appropriate thinking and behaviours, or by reducing their effects (coping).

ADAPTING TO STRESS

A young boy whose father continually shouts at him may just accept the fact, or adapt to it. If he sees other children experiencing the same kind of parental behaviour, he may assume that it is normal and the negative effects may be small. This is adapting to the stress.

The physical body and the mind can both make adaptations to stresses. The body may adjust by a reduced immune function that can result in a lower resistance to diseases and more frequent colds. Allergies causing asthma, acne or skin rashes may develop. The cardio-vascular system may react with higher blood pressure, tightness in the chest, or a heart that beats more rapidly or more strongly. The tension may cause increasing headaches. The muscular system can respond with pains in the back, neck or jaw. The gastro-intestinal system may be affected with symptoms of diarrhoea, constipation, burping, excess gas, or ulcers. The nervous system may show signs, such as dizziness, tics, menstrual irregularities, or sleep problems.

Psychologically, some people react with anger, boredom, depression, hopelessness, irritability, hostility, anxiety, panic, frustration, or fear. The method of adjustment is likely to be inherited, although some people 'learn' their adjustments by imitating others.

ELIMINATING STRESS AND REDUCING ITS EFFECTS

A number of measures can be taken to reduce the effects of the stressors, or to eliminate them. Many are the same as those activities which help health in every area of life – physical fitness, an effective sleep and relaxation regimen, sound nutrition, committed social relationships, a positive attitude towards life, meaningful life goals, and a knowledge of how to change behaviour for the better.

Effective adjustments to stress can only be made after determining whether or not it is indeed possible to do anything about that stress. If you want very badly to be on the first team in your club, but have not been selected, this is stressful. You might decide to work harder in order to make the team; you might decide to go to another club where you know you'll be selected; or you might give up the sport. You can fight, or you can flee from the stress. We are often faced with stressful situations to which we must adjust by non-action – a parking ticket, being fired, not being allowed to borrow the car, not being able to go skiing one weekend because of work pressures. Possible affirmative action might include asking for a transfer to another department, resigning from the job, or exercising to lessen the effects of pressures and stresses.

Exercise is often overlooked as an effective method of stress reduction; frequently, only its physiological benefits, and not its mental benefits, are recognized. It is, however, a known fact that forceful exercise, especially where hitting or kicking is involved, is an efficient way of reducing the effects of stress. Too often, stress is handled by reaching for tranquillizers, sleeping pills or alcohol, when there are far more effective solutions available.

What to Do

- Look for the causes of the stress. Can it be changed or must it be tolerated? Is it a person or a situation? Is the problem with you? Do other people react similarly to what you think is the cause of the problem?
- It is not necessary to win every confrontation. Evaluate your values and goals. Must some stresses be tolerated in order to accomplish a greater goal?
- Be positive. Too often, people concentrate on the negative aspects of a situation, looking at liabilities rather than assets, failures rather than successes. Successful adjustments require a positive approach.
- Seek advice. A friend or a professional counsellor may be able to give new insights, and will be able to relieve tensions. Talking over a problem is a tension-reliever.
- Do one thing at a time. The seconds quickly become minutes, hours, and years. When you concentrate on one thing at a time, you are more likely to be able to solve a stressful situation in a rational manner.
- Keep in mind that everyone is unique. Others people's problems are not necessarily exactly like yours. Similarities do exist, however, so it may be helpful to read what others have done in like situations or to attend a type of group therapy led by professionals.
- Train yourself to recognize an impending personal crisis. Emotional upsets at school or at work, arguments in marriage, and break-ups with people with whom we feel close, can initiate a mental problem.
- If you are uptight, anxiety-producing situations should be avoided. Societal problems on TV, violent movies or stress-filled family situations can accent our stresses. Take a holiday, go on a restful outing, or have a quiet time to lessen the feeling of anxiety.

COPING WITH STRESS

While the ideal way to handle unwanted stresses is to eliminate them, this is not always possible. Consequently, we must learn to handle the stresses, with coping skills, including relaxation techniques, exercise techniques, or diversion. Coping techniques, which may reduce the effects that distresses have on us, can be:

1. *cognitive* (from the mind to the body), such as meditation;
2. *somatic* (from the body to the mind), such as exercise; or
3. *behavioural approaches* (changing behaviours which are harmful), such as time management.

(Berger, Bonnie G., 'Coping with Stress: The effectiveness of exercise and other techniques', paper presented at the Annual Meeting of the American Academy of Kinesiology and Physical Education,

March 24, 1993, published in *Quest*, Vol. 46, 1994.)

Cognitive Techniques

Cognitive techniques begin with the mind. By correct thinking, or by 'non-thinking', the body can be relaxed and the tensions of the distresses reduced. Among the cognitive techniques are meditation, the relaxation response, hypnosis, and thought-stopping. Top-level athletes use these techniques as an essential part of their sport psychology training.

Meditation

Meditation is a type of non-thinking that the Hindus of India have used for thousands of years. During the 1960s, the Maharishi Mahesh Yogi came to the United States and both simplified and popularized the idea of meditation. The maharishi taught many people to teach his technique – repeating a mantra while breathing deeply, for fifteen to twenty minutes once or twice a day. Researchers at Stanford University, among others, proved that the techniques of the yogi reduced blood pressure and other symptoms of stress. (Feuerstein, M., Labbe, E.E., and Kuczmierczyk, A. R., *Health Psychology: A psychobiological perspective*, New York, Plenum, 1986, p. 189.) There is a very different set of physiological responses to meditation or the relaxation response from those to simple rest. (Dillbeck, M.C., Orme-Johnson, D.W., 'Physiological differences between transcendental meditation and rest', *American Psychologist*, Vol. 42, 1987, pp. 879–881.)

Dr Herbert Benson, a cardiologist at the Harvard Medical School, wrote in his book *The Relaxation Response* (William Morrow, New York, 1975) that meditation can be done by almost anyone, and that it doesn't have to be a religious experience.

He recommends achieving good relaxation as follows:

1. sit in a comfortable chair in a quiet room, assuming a restful position;
2. close your eyes, and try to relax all your muscles;
3. breathe through your nose, and become aware of and think about your breathing;
4. as you breathe out, say silently to yourself some one-syllable word that can free the mind from logical thought. You might use the word 'one' or 'on', or the Hindu word 'om' which is often used by yogis as a mantra. Don't use a word like 'sex' or 'money', as this will keep your mind active;
5. do this breathing, relaxing, and repetition of the word for about twenty minutes. You may open your eyes to check the clock, but it's important that you remain undisturbed for the entire period. Maintain a very passive attitude. Don't worry about how well you are meditating, or you may inhibit the response. If distracting thoughts occur, let them. The meditating word will return naturally.

This relaxation response of Dr Benson's has been extremely effective in lowering blood pressure. Many relaxation therapists say that it is impossible to be anxious or emotionally tense when you are relaxed. It has certainly been proven medically and psychologically that where there is anxiety there is muscle tension, and when muscle tension is relieved, so is the anxiety. Dr Benson believes that, with the stressful life that so many of us lead, we must do something to alleviate the damages of such a life. We should take relaxation breaks; avoid reaching for an artificial aid such as a cigarette, a drink, or a tranquilliser; perhaps take a nap during the day; use a meditation technique; or use a type of biofeedback.

The effects of relaxation on those with specific medical problems, such as high blood pressure and asthma, have been consistently demonstrated. At the Children's Memorial Hospital in Chicago, tests on eighty children between the ages of seven and fifteen found that all those who suffered repeated asthma attacks were able to subdue their attacks by learning to relax.

Meditation seems to work partly because it controls the *parasympathetic* nervous system. The nervous system is comprised of the *central* nervous system (the brain and spinal column), and the autonomic nervous system. The central nervous system is the thinking and feeling part, and the autonomic system regulates the arousal state. The autonomic system has two functions. The sympathetic system works when a person is nervous, controlling the 'fight or flight' reaction. The parasympathetic system works when the body is relaxed or asleep. When the sympathetic system is working, the blood pressure goes up, the heart beats more rapidly and the breathing is faster and shallow. When the parasympathetic system is working, the heart beats more slowly, the blood pressure is reduced, and the breathing is slow and deep.

By breathing slowly and deeply, the conscious mind (the central nervous system) can control one aspect of the parasympathetic system, and other physiological responses may follow, including lowered blood pressure and slow heart rate.

Hypnosis

In hypnosis, the mind is taught to relax through the power of suggestion. Some people are quite susceptible to such suggestion, while others are not. Hypnosis should only be done by a trained and licensed therapist.

Thought-Stopping

Thought-stopping is a technique in which unwanted stress-producing thoughts are removed. The individual imagines a situation in which the negative thoughts might occur – for example, taking an exam, missing a jump, or dealing with a discourteous customer at work. A timer is set for about three minutes of this imagining and, at the end, the therapist or the patient yells 'stop'. The individual then keeps his or her mind blank for about 30 seconds. If the thoughts return, the patient says 'stop'.

When the individual has been able to do this with the therapist's help, it is repeated without the therapist's intervention. At the third stage, positive and assertive thoughts are substituted for the undesired negative thoughts – 'I will relax during the second jump', or 'I am prepared for the second jump'. This method of 'thought-stopping' is often effective in eliminating obsessive stress-producing thinking, such as worrying.

Visualization

Mental imagery or visualization is a technique that is common among athletes. It involves imagining yourself – either from the outside, like watching yourself in a movie, or from the inside – doing what you want to do, or should do, in a certain situation. If you are trying to stop smoking after dinner, you may imagine yourself chewing gum or taking a walk at that time. Imagining the action can be influential in helping you perform it.

One way of improving sporting technique is to watch videos over and over again of sportspeople performing activities, such as skiing, perfectly. Your mind can learn how to ski better, and the proper muscles will actually contract as you visualize how you should be skiing. Top-level athletes have used such techniques for many years. Mental imagery is a very simple method of making positive changes to stressors. If you are a tennis player who has been hitting the ball too early, you might imagine yourself waiting for it to reach you before hitting.

Somatic Techniques

Somatic (body to mind) techniques are begun with the body as the focus, but the mind relaxes as the body responds to the specific technique. Among the somatic techniques are yoga, progressive relaxation, diaphragmatic breathing, massage, and physical exercise.

Yoga

Yoga is an ancient method of religious salvation of the Hindus, who had several yogas (paths) to religious experience. Hatha yoga, discussed here, is the method in which the body is controlled, usually by stretching and deep diaphragmatic breathing. The Hindu would use this as the starting point for mind control (meditation). Most people in the West use yoga as a relaxing and physical flex-ibility activity, gaining the ability to stretch tensed muscles and benefiting from the relaxation advantages of the breathing.

Many people do not use the diaphragm properly. They use the auxiliary breathing muscles of the chest and neck. Diaphragmatic breathing is deep breathing using the diaphragm (the major breathing muscle), and is a method of relaxation which is a part of many other techniques – meditation, relaxation response, progressive relaxation, yoga, swimming, and so on. The technique is useful because it does not require a great deal of practice and can be done anywhere and at any time.

Lie on the floor. Uncover the abdominal area so that you can see the skin between the lower part of the ribs and the hips. As you breathe, see that your abdomen is rising and falling. If your chest, but not your abdomen, is moving up and down, you are not using your diaphragm effectively.

Physical Exercise

Physical exercise can help relaxation in several ways. It can be a recreational pursuit, a rhythmic endurance exercise, or a pleasant physically fatiguing experience.

A recreational pursuit – a game of tennis or golf, a day of downhill skiing, or an afternoon of surfing or scuba diving – can make the participant forget about the problems which have created any stressful feelings.

A rhythmic activity – distance swimming, running, walking, or cross-country skiing – can provide both the diversion of a recreational activity and the rhythmic breathing of a meditation session. For such an exercise to have stress-reducing effects, the following must be true:

1. it should be enjoyable;
2. it should be aerobic and should not be considered to be competitive by the participant;
3. it should be of moderate intensity and last at least twenty minutes. (Berger, Bonnie, 'Mood Alteration with Exercise: A taxonomy to maximize benefits', paper presented at the VIII World Congress of Sport Psychology, Lisbon, Portugal, June 23, 1993.)

While people generally report that they feel better after exercise, not all exercise is equally beneficial. In fact, some participants in exercise have been seen to suffer an *increase* in stress: a competitive runner or swimmer working to exhaustion so that a peak performance can be achieved in the championships; recreational swimmers swimming in uncomfortably warm water; a golfer or tennis player under pressure to win.

Those who are particularly competitive in their recreational pursuits may negate the potential stress-reducing benefits. If exercise is to be used to reduce stress, it must be pleasant; it must be 'play'. Running may be play for one person but work for another. Shooting baskets may be play, but taking part in the recreational league championship may be distressful – especially if you are losing.

Many people have experienced a particularly high level of stress relief after 30 to 50 minutes of aerobic activity. This is often called the 'exercise high' and may be related to the brain's reaction to increased endorphins (brain chemicals similar to opium).

Participating in exercise (particularly aerobic exercise) several times a week for more than a year, shows greater psychological benefits. It has been found that in a runner who had run at least thirty miles a week for two years, a single episode of high-intensity work on a treadmill greatly reduces the anxiety level and increases the alpha brain waves (those present during meditation). However, the same episode of exercise did not produce these same levels of relaxation in people who were not long-time runners. (Boutcher, S.H. and Landers, D. M., 'The effects of vigorous exercise on anxiety, heart rate, and alpha activity of runners and non runners', *Psychophysiology*, Vol. 25, 1988, pp. 696–702.) These stress reduction benefits increased as the number of exercise sessions per week and the number of weeks increased. The benefits from the exercise seem to last two to four hours. (Raglin, J.S. and Morgan, W.P., 'Influences of exercise and quiet rest on state anxiety and blood pressure', *Medicine and Science in Sports and Exercise*, Vol. 19, 1987, pp. 436–463.)

A person who is physically fit will usually have a better self-concept and self esteem than one who is unfit, and should therefore be better able to handle stressors. (Tucker, L.A., 'Effect of weight training on body attitudes: who benefits most?', *Journal of Sports Medicine and Physical Fitness*, Vol. 27, 1987, pp. 70–78; Young, M. L., 'Estimation of fitness and physical ability, physical performance, and self-concept among adolescent females', *Journal of Sports Medicine and Physical Fitness*, Vol. 25, 1985, pp. 144–150.) Exercise activities that have a positive outcome are more likely to result in a better self-concept. The positive outcome might be:

1. success (such as running or swimming faster, or losing weight and developing a more pleasing body shape),
2. increased feeling of physical competence (such as skiing or playing tennis better); or
3. goal attainment (such as lifting a heavier weight, reducing resting pulse rate, or shooting a lower golf score).

Effective exercise has also been shown to reduce the illnesses that often accompany stressful events in life. (Brown, J.D., 'Staying fit and staying well: physical fitness as a moderator of life stress', *Journal of Personality and Social Psychology*, Vol. 60, 1991, pp. 555–561). Exercisers report a lower incidence of colon, breast, and prostate cancer. (Mackinnon, L. T., 'Exercise and immunology: current issues in exercise science', Monograph No. 2; Champaign, I.L., *Human Kinetics*, 1992; Sternfeld, B., 'Cancer and the protective effect of physical activity: the epidemiological evidence', *Medicine and Science in Sports and Exercise*, Vol. 24, 1991, pp. 1195–1209.)

Exercise is both an effective method of preventing the stronger negative reactions that can result from stressors, and a way of reducing those negative reactions when they are present. It has been shown to be as effective as other stress management techniques in reducing depression, tension, and anger. (Berger, B.G., Friedman, E. and Easton, M., 'Comparison of jogging, the relaxation response, and group interaction for stress reduction', *Journal of Sport and Exercise Psychology*, Vol. 10, 1988, pp. 431–447; Long, B.C. and Haney, C.J., 'Coping strategies for working women: aerobic exercise and relaxation interventions', *Behavior Therapy*, Vol. 19, 1988, pp. 75–83; Long and Haney, 'Long-term follow-up of stressed working women: a comparison of aerobic exercise and progressive relaxation', *Journal of Sport and Exercise Psychology*, Vol. 10, 1988, pp. 461–470.) Exercising aerobically is inexpensive and takes the same amount of time as other techniques, while offering many additional benefits, so it should be high on everyone's list of daily activities.

Choosing a Coping Technique

Stress may be more effectively handled by choosing an appropriate coping technique:

1. if symptoms are physical – tense muscles, a rapid heart rate, or a lack of energy – a physical activity may be the best way of handling the stress; try running, swimming, cycling, cross-country skiing, massage, or yoga for stress reduction;

2. if stress reactions are mental – anxiety, worry, insomnia, and negative thinking – the better choices for coping may be meditation, the relaxation response, or hypnosis;

3. for stresses caused by a hectic schedule, having too many things to do and too much responsibility, try assertiveness training (to be able to say 'no'), time management (to be better at scheduling the important activities), biofeedback, and psychological assistance to change to a more relaxed way of living.

REDUCING OR ELIMINATING DISTRESSES

The ideal method for handling stresses is to eliminate them, if that is a possibility. Effective thinking can help in this area, and will also help to raise self-esteem, because it is an important aspect of our self-evaluation. Effective decision-making is the sign of a mature person. But what are the steps to effective thinking and effective problem-solving? How can everyone use the proven thinking techniques to reduce or eliminate problems and stresses in life?

The Scientific Method of Problem Solving

American philosopher-psychologist-educator John Dewey can be credited with the following approach to solving problems. He believed that the method of science can be applied to individual problems; and that, when applied, it should make the problems more easily soluble. Here are the steps that might be used to solve a problem:

1. define the problem;
2. clarify the problem with facts about it;
3. look at several possible solutions;
4. choose the best possible solution;
5. try it and evaluate its outcome.

Successful use of problem-solving can reduce stresses at every age and can even reduce severe depression ('The Menninger Letter', June 1994, p. 6). It takes thought, time, and commitment to the above steps.

Defining the problem may be more difficult than it seems. Many problems are simple, but others are more complex and need to be broken down into component problems, each of which is then capable of solution. Included in the definition of the problem is the question, 'How do I know it is really a problem?' Do you have evidence that you are too fat? Has a doctor told you? Or do you just want to diet because losing weight is fashionable?

Clarifying the problem is the second, key step in problem-solving. Get some facts about your problem from talking to an expert – a doctor or psychologist – or reading books in the library, current periodicals, or a computer database. Get a better understanding about whether it should be of immediate concern, or whether it is as serious as you think. You may find out what

measures to take to solve the problem, or gain some insight into it.

For example, if you plan to diet, look at the major approaches to losing weight – eating smaller portions, reducing the percentage of fat, increasing fibres, reducing alcohol and other empty calories, burning off calories through exercise.

Possible solutions must be based on the facts and opinions that you have researched. If you want to diet, and you have researched the subject, you will have several alternatives from which to choose, and will know the advantages and disadvantages of each method of weight loss.

Choose the best solution or solutions from the alternatives. You might have come up with ten possible solutions to your weight problem. From these solutions you might select: lowering the number of calories consumed each day by 300; cutting down a little bit on all the foods you consume; and starting an exercise programme.

Test the solution, by trying it out for a week or two. If it works, you are on the way to solving the problem. If it doesn't, you will need to try other possible solutions.

Decision-Making

Making decisions is often difficult for people, because it forces them to take the initiative to think. A French naturalist conducted an experiment in which he placed several caterpillars on the rim of a flowerpot. They followed each other around the rim for seven days and nights until they all died of starvation, even though plenty of food was available in the pot. Too often, we behave like these caterpillars, and follow the lead of others. However, our best chance of making our life satisfying and happy is to take the time to work through problems and to choose effectively.

Every choice is a chance. Living is a risk, and every new course of action has its uncertainties. Perhaps fear too often stifles our thinking.

The best method to use when stresses occur is to think through the problem, and then try to eliminate the negative stressor. It may mean changing jobs; it may mean finding another place to live; for the sportsperson, it may mean lowering his or her level of competition.

PAIN

Every athlete experiences pain at some time. It may be the kick in the shin for a football player, agony in the thighs for a rower as the finish line approaches, or 'hitting the wall' in a marathon. The capacity to handle pain depends on a number of factors – previous pain experiences, cultural backgrounds, or the way the nervous system is set up to transmit the pain.

Everyone has certain 'pain beliefs'. Some believe that their pain will last a long time, while others, with exactly the same pain, believe that that pain will be short-lived. Part of a person's pain belief system ascribes blame for the pain either to him or herself, or to other factors, such as fate. If responsibility for the pain is taken on, the person has control over it. If other factors are blamed, it is hard to believe that much can be done about the pain.

Anxiety can also increase pain. It has been found that dental patients who experienced pain during their last visit to the dentist were more likely to be anxious, and expect pain, on a subsequent visit. Similarly, an athlete who over-estimates the severity of an injury tends to experience more pain.

Athletes realize that their activities increase their chance of injury. The choice of sport may be determined by the chance of injury. Those prepared to take more risk may opt for football or downhill skiing, while lower-risk takers may choose running or cross-country skiing. That choice may be associated with a higher pain tolerance and less fear of injury among those inclined to take more risk. Studies in the United States have shown that American football players have a greater tolerance for pain than karate or fencing participants.

Athletes tend to believe that injury will heal quickly, but those who are actually injured adjust their expectations. The essential understanding must be that everyone is in control of his or her body, and this goes a long way in making the injured person do the right things to get well. Educated people have been found generally to report less pain, and this may be because they see themselves as the cause and as the cure of the pain.

For the athlete who believes him or herself to be in control of the pain, the advice of a doctor or physical therapist, and therapy itself can aid a speedy recovery. Those who don't believe they have control will tend to skip their therapy and therefore prolong the recovery time.

BEING IN CONTROL

In the area of developing psychological improvement and outlook – in sport or in other aspects of daily life – the way we see problems, and the way we see ourselves as being able to develop solutions to problems, is critical. We must feel that we are in control. Perhaps the most succinct reflection of this task came from the German theologian

Reinhold Niebuhr, in what is called 'The Serenity Prayer':

'God grant me -

the *serenity* to accept the things I cannot change;

the *courage* to change the things I can; and

the *wisdom* to know the difference.'

CHAPTER 17
Over-Training

OVER-TRAINING SYNDROME

John Dryden said, 'The wise, for cure, on exercise depend.' However, some people exercise excessively and can develop health problems as a result of a heavy work schedule. There is no question that effective endurance exercise is a great benefit to health – it reduces high blood pressure, it reduces heart attack risk, it reduces the risk of some cancers, and builds up immunity to fight off other diseases. There are times, however, when the body gets too much exercise, and the body or the mind cannot recover from it. While usually temporary and reversible, the possible negative outcome of physical or mental stress from exercise must be taken into account.

Symptoms

The negative effects are most likely to happen to elite athletes, or to recreational exercisers who train far more than normal. Those who train excessively usually participate in the endurance sports, and suffer from what is called 'over-training syndrome' or 'chronic fatigue syndrome'. It has also been called 'staleness' or 'burn-out'. The symptoms are primarily fatigue and under-performance, and may include a loss of motivation, increased injuries or illnesses, loss of appetite, loss of body weight, irritability or other mood changes, depression, insomnia, nightmares, a loss of sex drive (libido). Women can also develop menstrual problems (*see* Chapter 18). Any one of these

symptoms can be an indication of the effects of over-training. If the athlete does not recover after two weeks of rest, then the over-training syndrome could be said to exist.

Occurrence of the Syndrome

The over-training syndrome is generally thought to be more likely to occur in men running over 40 miles (60km) a week, or in women running over 30 miles (45km) a week (Pate, Russell, in a symposium on elite athletes held at the Pre-Olympic Scientific Congress at Dallas, Texas, July 11, 1996). However, others have found the level to be as high as 100 miles (150km) a week (Kuipers, H., 'How much is too much? Performance aspects of over-training', Pre-Olympic Scientific Congress, Dallas, Texas, July 13, 1996.)

Athletes often think that increasing the workout will bring increased results. This isn't always true. In one study, doubling a swimming workout actually reduced the performance of the swimmers. In speed skating it has been found that practising more than fifteen hours a week is counter-productive. A competitive athlete needs to judge workouts, so that they maximize performance, and don't lead to over-training and a reduction in competitive abilities.

Over-training is common at the beginning of a sports season, particularly if the athlete has engaged in interval training – short intense bouts of exercise for one to five minutes each. Long-distance monotonous training can also be a factor. Varied workouts are more likely to keep the athlete's psychological spirits up.

Ten per cent of the elite college swimmers in the United States have suffered some symptoms of the over-training syndrome. It is not uncommon for them to swim four to six miles (6-9km) twice a day during the season, and coaches will generally 'taper' the workouts as championship meets approach. During the tapered part of the programme, there is more sprinting and they swim far less distance in total. One researcher in the USA has also monitored the moods of swimmers. If their moods were 'up', they were given more work, if they were low, their workload was reduced. This seems to indicate that the mood of an athlete is somewhat predictive of the onset of the over-training syndrome.

Poor nutrition is a common cause of several problems related to over-training, and the female athlete triad (*see* Chapter 18). The major problem is generally that there are insufficient calories to replace those being used in training. Since appetite is often reduced after training, many people do not take in enough calories, even if they are consuming more than someone on a normal diet.

Effects

The effects of over-training or chronic fatigue can be:
1. *mechanical* – stressing of bones (including stress fractures), ligaments, muscles and tendons;
2. *metabolic* – depletion of carbohydrates; inadequate amounts of adenosine triphosphate (ATP), essential in the release of energy in the muscles; excess of stress-related hormones (particularly cortisol); reduced resistance to infections, and so on;
3. *systemic* – involving the whole body or the mind–body relationship, including mental staleness and general tiredness.

What to Do

The amount of time needed to recover varies with the problem. Bones and tendons take longer to recover than muscles. Replenishing carbohydrates may take only a day or two but mental staleness may take some time. Effectiveness and speed of recovery depend on several factors – age, physiological make-up, the altitude at which the person is exercising, the temperature, and the athlete's physical condition.

Anyone who believes they may be suffering from the over-training syndrome, because of symptoms of excess tiredness or poor performance, should see their doctor. The symptoms may be caused by something other than over-training – perhaps psychological problems related to home, school or work; or physiological problems related to drugs or alcohol.

Prevention

The major preventive approach is to individualize training so that over-tiredness does not occur. Planned rests to allow recovery must be part of the training programme. Hard and light training on alternate days can be very effective.

Basic nutritional needs must be met. The athlete must consume enough carbohydrate, protein, fat, and water, as well as an adequate amount of vitamins and minerals (*see* Chapters 19 and 20). Carbohydrates must be replaced in the muscles because they are the major fuel in aerobic exercise.

Branched chain amino acids (BCAA) increase the amount of glutamine available to the immune system. For this reason, BCAA may need to be supplemented in the diet of an endurance athlete. If laboratory tests show low iron stores, the doctor may prescribe iron supplementation. There is no evidence that extra vitamin or mineral supplements will help an athlete avoid the over-training syndrome, although they may reduce the effects of osteoporosis.

Adequate rest is essential. Some people need well over ten hours of sleep a night, while others can survive on just a few hours. Heavy exercisers generally need more than the average person. Remember, the over-training syndrome is sometimes called the 'under-recovery syndrome'.

Psychological factors are often part of the problem, reducing the athlete's tolerance either to the physical demands of exercise, or to the psychological demands of competition. When psychological factors are involved, counselling, relaxation techniques, massage, and other stress reduction approaches may be useful (*see* Chapter 16).

REDUCED IMMUNITY

The immune system can be affected by over-training, and colds and other minor infections may become more common. This may be because of a reduction of glutamine, one of the non-essential amino acids. (It is called 'non-essential' because it need not be consumed every day, unlike 'essential' amino acids; if it is not consumed, it is made from other amino acids.) Glutamine is, however, essential to the body's functioning (*see* Chapter 19, on nutrition), as a fuel for the cells of the immune system. While it is normally released by the body's muscles, its release is reduced by endurance exercise.

Another factor which may be related to the reduced immune function is higher levels of cortisol, a hormone released when the body is stressed. This reduces several types of white blood cells that are disease fighters. After three hours of running, the cortisol level is doubled or tripled, and it stays elevated for about twelve hours.

The cancer-killing 'killer cells' in the body are reduced by as much as 50 per cent as the body ages, a major reason for the increase in cancers later in life. The running of a marathon reduces these cells, but they do return to normal or higher levels within a few days. More importantly, the positive effect of running increases these cells for long-distance runners when they are resting, or running less than 10 miles (15km) a day.

In a study done at a recent Los Angeles Marathon it was found that among those who ran the race, 14 per cent soon developed upper respiratory infections. Among those who signed up for the race, but did not run, only 2 per cent developed such problems. It is reasonable to assume that both groups were similarly trained, and that the actual running of the marathon reduced the immunity (Neiman, David, Symposium on elite athletes, Pre-Olympic Scientific Congress, Dallas, Texas, July 11, 1996). The increase in infections seems to occur in people running more than 60 miles (90km) a week. This would be approximately equivalent to swimming 15 miles (25km) a week or cycling 150 miles (225km) a week.

To reduce the chance of becoming ill:
1. make sure that you get enough sleep;
2. allow recovery from hard training;
3. get enough food, particularly carbohydrates and vitamin C;
4. have annual flu shots.

CHAPTER 18
The Female Athlete

THE FEMALE ATHLETE TRIAD

(We are indebted to Dr Barbara Drinkwater of the Pacific Medical Center in Seattle, Washington, and former president of the American College of Sports Medicine, for her input on this section.)

Female endurance athletes, gymnasts, figure skaters and dancers are often afflicted by one (or a combination) of three major problems:
1. eating disorders (*anorexia* or *bulimia*);
2. *amenorrhoea* (no menstruation), or *oligomenorrhoea* (little menstruation);
3. *osteoporosis* (a loss of bone minerals, particularly calcium, resulting in weakened bones).

EATING PROBLEMS

Occurrence

Dancers and gymnasts are most likely to have eating problems because of a pressure to keep their weight excessively low. The highest incidence is found among women and girls who participate in 'aesthetic' sports, such as gymnastics and dancing; from 35 to more than 60 per cent of gymnasts have eating problems. Endurance athletes, such as swimmers and marathon runners, may also develop the same kind of problems because they are not replacing the calories lost during training. Studies have shown that as many as 15 to 27 per cent of female competitive swimmers and long-distance runners

may have eating problems. A Norwegian study showed that 33 per cent of their elite cross-country skiers were affected. The problem is much more prevalent among athletes in individual sports than in team sports.

Eating patterns among physically active women range from normal, through inadequate, to the severely neurotic states of advanced anorexia or bulimia. A low nutritional intake will almost certainly affect menstrual patterns and, once this happens, bone loss is almost certain to occur. (Nattiv, Aurelia; Drinkwater, Barbara, *et al.*, 'The female athletic triad', *Clinics in Sports Medicine: The Athletic Woman*, W.B. Saunders, 13:2, April 1994, pp. 405–418.)

Anorexia nervosa

Anorexia nervosa is a disease primarily seen in young women; it involves a psychological fear of food and any weight gain, resulting in 'voluntary' starvation. It afflicts nearly one in one hundred women (Balaa, M.A. and Drossman, D.A., 'Anorexia Nervosa and Bulimia: The eating disorders', *Disease of the Month*, Year Book Medical Publishers, Chicago, June 1985, pp. 1–52), although 5 to 10 per cent of its victims are male.

The sufferer with this disease goes on a diet and refuses to stop, no matter how much weight is lost. They may take up, or increase participation in, endurance sports to bring about even more weight loss; at first, performance may be good, but it quickly deteriorates as there is not enough fuel for training. The disease has a psychological basis, but its physical effects are very real, and medical care, usually hospitalization, is generally required. About one in ten of those who have this affliction starve themselves to death.

There may be a hereditary pre-disposition to anorexia. Identical twins exhibit the disease four to five times more often than non-identical twins do. However, Western culture, with the high value it places on thinness, almost certainly contributes. Parents who value outward appearance and social achievement in a child, rather than self-esteem and self-actualization, are often associated with the anorexic person (Whitney, Eleanor, and Hamilton, Eva, *Understanding Nutrition,* West Publishing, 1987, p. 281), as is an absent or distant father.

Once the anorexic has begun the severe dieting routine, symptoms of starvation may set in, leading to a number of physical problems. The physical effects may include the following:

- abnormal thyroid, adrenal, and growth hormone functions;
- a weakened heart muscle;
- amenorrhoea, due to the low percentage of body fat;
- a drop in blood pressure;
- anaemia, due to the lack of protein and iron ingested;
- a slowing of the peristalsis of the intestines;
- atrophying of the lining of the intestines;
- inability of the pancreas to secrete many of its enzymes;
- a drop in body temperature;
- a drying of the skin;
- an increase of body hair as the body tries to keep itself warm;

- the worst possible effect of the disease is death.

Because dieting is so common in western society, anorexia can be difficult to diagnose until its advanced stages have been entered. However, other symptoms – moodiness, being withdrawn, seeming to have an obsession about food but not being seen eating it, and constant food preparation – may be observed by those close to the anorexic. Once the disease has been diagnosed, a number of medical and psychological therapies can be effective.

Bulimia

Bulimia, or *bulimia nervosa,* is more common than anorexia. Typically, the sufferer restricts calorie intake during the day and binges on high-fat, high-calorie foods at least twice a week. Following the binge, the person will then purge, in an attempt to rid the body of the excess calories, by vomiting, using laxatives, fasting, or doing an excessive amount of exercise. Some experts do not consider behaviour to be 'bulimic' until it has persisted for about three months, with two or more binges per week. Estimates based on various surveys of college students and others indicate that between 5 and 20 per cent of women may be bulimic. It is also more common among men than anorexia is.

Bulimia, like anorexia, stems from a psychological problem. However there may also be a link to physical abnormalities in some cases. The neurotransmitters serotonin and norepinephrine seem to be involved, as does the hormone cholecystokinin; this hormone is secreted by the hypothalamus, and makes a person feel that enough food has been eaten.

Physical symptoms that may be seen depend on the type of purging technique used. The bulimic who induces vomiting can have scars on the back of the knuckles, mouth sores, gingivitis, tooth decay, a swollen oesophagus, and chronic bad breath. The bulimic who uses laxatives can cause irreparable damage to the intestines due to constant diarrhoea. All bulimics run the risk of throwing off electrolytes (minerals involved in muscle contractions) due to constant dehydration. This imbalance of electrolytes can cause the bulimic to have abnormal heart rhythms, and can induce a heart attack.

Anorexia and bulimia affect 10 to 20 per cent of teenage and young adult females. In some sports, the incidence can be much higher, either because a thin body is an advantage, or because a stressful aerobic training programme requires more calories than the athlete is willing to consume. Gymnastics, diving and cheer-leading are examples of the first type, distance running and swimming are examples of the second type, and figure skating or dancing (ballet, modern, jazz) can be a combination of the two.

Women need much more iron than men do, and iron supplementation is advisable. Calcium supplementation is advised if calcium is not adequately available in the diet, and vitamin D may also be needed, because it aids in the hardening of the bones.

Anorexia athletica

Anorexia athletica is the athletic version of *anorexia nervosa*. It is an intense fear of gaining weight, even though the athlete is generally at least 5 per cent less than the expected weight for her age and height. The victims may eat less, as in *anorexia nervosa*, and purge through vomiting, laxatives, and/or diuretics, as in bulimia. They may also binge eat. Additionally, they exercise compulsively to use up at least as many calories as they have consumed. (Sundgot-Borgen, J and Larsen, S., 'Nutrition intake and eating behavior of female elite athletes suffering from *anorexia nervosa, anorexia athletica,* and *bulimia nervosa'*, *International Journal of Sport Nutrition*, 3:431–442, 1993; also Sundgot-Borgen, J., presentation 'The Female Athlete Triad', at European Women and Sport Conference, Stockholm, Sweden, August 24, 1996.)

OVER-EXERCISING

Some researchers have expressed the belief that as many as 75 per cent of anorexia cases may begin with over-exercising. A high volume of exercise not only uses calories but also often suppresses the desire to eat. This may be because of an increase in endorphins, the naturally-occurring opium-like compounds in the brain that make us feel good. Endorphins are often increased by 'good' activities, such as exercise and listening to classical music, and they can be decreased by such activities as taking illegal drugs and listening to loud rock music.

MENSTRUAL PROBLEMS

Menstrual problems in athletes occur primarily because of insufficient calorie intake. It can be insufficient either because of an eating disorder, or because calories used during the exercise period are not being replaced, even though meals consumed might be adequate for a non-exercising woman. The stress of training and competition can also play a part.

The average age for the first menstrual cycle is twelve and a half, but serious dancers and competitive gymnasts, figure skaters, runners and swimmers begin menstruating on average about two and a half years later. Many who begin their athletic careers later will stop or have infrequent menses. It is essential to keep menstruation normal to avoid bone damage. Generally, the cycle returns to normal within two to three months of reducing a training regimen, and obtaining adequate nutrition.

Amenorrhoea is often related to a reduction of oestrogen, the major female hormone. Oestrogen levels of most amenorrhoeic women are similar to those women who have entered menopause. Another factor affecting menstruation is the reduction of the luteinizing hormone (LH), which is necessary to complete the menstrual cycle. It can be reduced either by an excess of exercise, or by a diet too low in calories for the work being done. (Loucks, A., Symposium of elite athletes, Pre-Olympic Scientific Congress, Dallas, Texas, July 11, 1996.) Girls and women who have a heavy exercise programme must eat enough, if they wish to reduce the risk of the female athlete triad. With adequate food intake, the athlete's menstrual cycle can remain normal. For example, 60 per cent of the runners in the New York Marathon report normal menstrual cycles.

EXERCISE DURING MENSTRUATION

Women generally become stronger during menstruation. Their hand strength and jumping ability are increased and, according to many world record holders, many records are set during menstruation.

(We are indebted to Dr Karin Henriksson-Larsen, MD of the University of Umeå, Sweden, for her input in this area, in which she has done important research.)

OSTEOPOROSIS

Causes and Occurrence

Osteoporosis is almost certain to occur when amenorrhoea occurs. Women in developed countries are likely to have their maximum mineral content in their bones during their teenage years. However, teenage endurance athletes and dancers often have very low bone density and can be likened to 70-year-old women in this respect. Both the lack of oestrogen, leading to amenorrhoea, and the lack of nutrients, due to inadequate food intake, contribute to the lack of bone minerals.

Some of the bone loss may be irreversible. The loss of the bone material puts the athlete at increased risk of broken bones. Stress fractures are more easily developed, as are fractures of the pelvis, hip and spine.

Prevention

Assuming that an athlete's diet is adequate, bone density can be increased by weight training and weight-bearing exercise. When the bones are subjected to stress, they become stronger. This is particularly important to women who swim – swimming does not stress the bones, since the water supports the body. Runners get some help from their weight-bearing activities, and rowers from the stress on the spine but, although this lessens the bone-thinning effect, it does not eliminate it. Their exercise offers limited protection, only of the stressed bones, so

143

rowers' hips and runners' wrists, for example, have no protection. The use of resistance exercises in the gym or at home will help.

In one study it was found that female runners who ran more miles per week had more fractures. The unanswered question, however, was whether these resulted from bone loss, or from over-training and over-stressing the bones through constant pounding on the ground. Another study found that female rowers who did not menstruate had only 9 per cent less bone density than other rowers who were menstruating regularly. This figure was less than expected; it is possible that the stress on the bones from rowing has a strengthening effect that somewhat counteracts the negative effects of the lack of menstruation.

Male Symptoms

Some male athletes, including competitive wrestlers, lightweight rowers, judo competitors, jockeys, weight-lifters and boxers, need to reduce their body weight. Some endurance athletes, such as marathon runners, may have a food intake that is lower than desirable. These athletes may all suffer similar symptoms to females who experience the female triad. In men, the symptoms are more likely to be reduced bone mass and increased susceptibility to stress fractures, low testosterone (the sex hormone), with a lower sperm count, and weight loss through taking in insufficient calories.

What to Do
To reduce the chance of developing osteoporosis:
1. consume adequate calcium – 1200mg daily;
2. consume adequate vitamin D – 400 iu;
3. have adequate manganese (300mg), zinc (12mg) and copper (2mg) in the daily diet;
4. do weight-bearing activities such as walking, running or strength training.

STRENGTH

The average woman has about 70 per cent of the lower body strength of a man, and about 50 per cent of the upper body strength. Women generally have the same strength per square centimetre of the cross-section of the muscle fibre as men; they just have fewer and smaller fibres. Strength training increases the size of the type 2 (fast twitch) muscle fibres more than the size of the type 1 (slow twitch endurance) muscle fibres.

ENDURANCE

Women in general have only about 70 per cent of the endurance capacity of men, due primarily to their smaller body size; however, their capacity for endurance work is only about 5 per cent less after the effect of the greater amount of body fat is considered. A woman can work for a longer time before exhaustion, probably because of the higher energy yield from her body fat. The female hormone *oestradiol* makes it easier for a woman to use fat for energy than a man.

On the other hand, men have about 6 per cent more red blood cells, which carry the oxygen. Their oxygen-carrying capacity is about 15 per cent higher than that of a woman. This means that a woman's heart must beat faster to get the oxygen to the muscles (assuming that the man and the woman are the same size).

A woman's anaerobic capacity (the ability to work without the use of the air breathed in) is about 15 per cent less than that of a man. This means that women must rely on air breathed in earlier in their competition. Men use up their anaerobic potentials after they have run about 1 mile (1500m), while women deplete their anaerobic reserves at about half a mile (800m).

OTHER CONCERNS FOR WOMEN

Female athletes are more likely than males to suffer leg problems. Less dense bones, wider hips with the resulting increased leg angles, and looser ligaments may all contribute to the increased risk. Physical activity can promote better health, as long as adequate food intake is continued. Weight-bearing activities such as walking and running increase bone density, and can reverse osteoporosis.

THE PREGNANT ATHLETE

The majority of women should be able to begin or continue an exercise programme during pregnancy. A doctor should be consulted, however, because there are several factors which may make aerobic exercise inadvisable – these may include vaginal bleeding, poorly controlled diabetes, kidney disease, heart disease, high blood pressure, very low body weight, and multiple pregnancy. Smoking and alcohol consumption should always be stopped during pregnancy, but this becomes even more important in an exercising woman, when even less oxygen can get to the brain of the foetus.

SYMPTOMS OF ANOREXIA NERVOSA

Physical
- Weight 15 per cent below what is expected
- Amenorrhoea
- Dehydration
- Excessive fatigue
- Gastro-intestinal problems (constipation, diarrhoea, bloating)
- Feeling cold
- Being hyperactive

Psychological
- Intense fear of becoming overweight
- 'Feeling fat', even when very thin
- Avoidance of eating or eating situations
- Anxiety
- Unusual weighing habits (refusal to weigh, excessive weighing)
- Restlessness
- Depression or insomnia
- Compulsiveness about eating or exercising habits.

SYMPTOMS OF BULIMIA NERVOSA

Physical
- Purging (vomiting, using laxatives, etc.)
- Abrasion on back of hand from induced vomiting
- Dehydration
- Dental and gum problems
- Low weight, despite eating a great deal
- Menstrual irregularity
- Muscle cramps or weakness
- Gastro-intestinal problems
- Use of laxatives or diuretics beyond that prescribed by a doctor

Psychological
- Secret binge eating (at least twice a week for 3 or more months)
- A lack of control over eating
- Too much concern with body shape
- Depression
- Unnecessary dieting
- Excessive exercise beyond what is required for the sport
- Disappearing after eating (to toilet)

Symptoms of Amenorrhoea
- 'Primary amenorrhoea' means not having had a menstrual period by 16 years of age.
- 'Secondary amenorrhoea' means the stopping of menstrual periods once a girl or woman has begun menstruating; no periods for 3 to 6 consecutive months.
- 'Oligomenorrhoea' means a very long time between menstrual flows, with a total cycle of 35 to 90 days.

CHAPTER 19
Basics of Nutrition

BASIC UNDERSTANDING

A basic understanding of the science of nutrition, and the ability to develop a proper diet, is essential to healthy living. It is especially important for people involved in sports to understand what nutrients they need, for their general health, for their sporting performance, and for the prevention of injury, disease and illness. Furthermore, certain dietary tools are necessary if the body is to recover quickly from injury or illness.

The scientific knowledge of nutrition doubles about every three years. Unfortunately, very few of people, athletes included, consume even the minimum amount of each of the necessary nutrients – protein, fat, carbohydrates, vitamins, and minerals – or of the essential 'non-nutrients' of fibre and water.

Protein, fat and carbohydrates bring with them the energy required to keep the body alive, as well as their specific contributions. All the food energy we consume comes in the form of calories. Vitamins, minerals, fibre and water do not bring with them calories when consumed.

CALORIES

The 'calorie' used in counting food energy is really a [kilojoule] kilocalorie. In one [kilojoule] kilocalorie, there is enough energy to heat 1kg of water by 1 degree centigrade (or two quarts of water by one and three-quarter degrees Fahrenheit; or to lift 3,000lb of weight one foot high).

Most people need about 10 calories per pound of body weight each day just to stay alive. If there is any physical activity at all, the body may need about 17 calories per pound per day in order to keep going. The starvation level for the average person is around 1200 calories per day, but anyone doing regular exercise will use many more.

PROTEIN

Protein is made up of twenty-two amino acids, otherwise known as the 'building blocks of life'. Amino acids are made up of carbon, hydrogen, oxygen, and nitrogen. While both fats and carbohydrates contain the first three elements, nitrogen is found only in protein. Protein is essential for building nearly every part of the body – the brain, heart, organs, skin, muscles, and even the blood.

Requirements

There are four calories in one gram of protein. Adults require 0.75g of protein per kg of body weight per day, or one-third of a gram of protein per pound, or just under 5g per stone. An easy way to estimate protein requirements in grams per day is to divide the body weight in pounds by 3. Anyone who weighs 150 pounds (10 stone 10 pounds) would need about 50g of protein per day. Children need 1.15g of protein per kg of body weight. This translates into about half a gram of protein per pound, so an easy way to determine the number of grams required per day is to divide the child's weight in pounds by 2. The elderly may require as much protein a day as children, due to their decreased energy intake, coupled with a possible decreased utilization of dietary protein.

Physically active adults have been thought to require more protein than is recommended by the United States Recommended Daily Allowance (USRDA), which is set at 0.8g per kg of body weight per day. In fact, most active people need not eat additional protein if they keep 12–15 per cent of their total calories as protein. Since active individuals need to consume more calories per day than their inactive counterparts, due to their increased energy expenditure, active adults who keep their protein intake at around 15 per cent of their total calories will eat more protein per day and thereby fulfil their body's protein requirement. Excess protein consumption (above the body's requirement) will be broken down, and the calories will either be burned off or stored as fat.

The athlete involved in a strenuous strength training regimen may need to increase the protein intake percentage, depending on the amount of total calories consumed per day. Strength-trained athletes have been shown to adapt to diets considered low in protein (0.86g per kg per day) by decreasing the amount of protein they use for muscle building. However, those who participate in heavy resistance training may choose to follow a diet higher in protein (1.4g per kg per day), to elicit maximum benefit from their workouts. This increased protein demand also appears true for body-builders who train intensively (one and a half hours per day, six days per week).

Amino Acids

In order to build tissues – organs, muscles, and blood – the body must have all of the necessary amino acids. The body can manufacture some of them – known as the non-essential amino acids – while others (the essential amino acids) must be obtained from food. During childhood, nine of the twenty-two amino acids are essential, but the adult body generally acquires the ability to synthesize one additional amino acid (*histidine*). This means that the adult body needs to find eight essential amino acids in the food consumed daily.

Amino acids cannot be stored in the body, and the minimum amounts of protein must therefore be consumed every day. If adequate protein is not consumed, the body immediately begins to break down tissue (usually beginning with muscle tissue) to release the essential amino acids. If even one essential amino acid is lacking, the other essential ones are not able to work to their full capacity. For example, if *methionine* (the most commonly lacking amino acid) is present at 60 per cent of the minimum requirement, the other seven essential amino acids are limited to near to 60 per cent of their potential. When they are not used, amino acids are deaminated, and excreted as urea in the urine.

Protein Sources

Animal products (fish, poultry, beef) and animal by-products (milk, eggs, cheese) are rich in readily usable protein. When animal products or by-products are eaten, their protein can be converted into protein in the body, because these sources have all of the essential amino acids in a proportion similar to that needed by humans. These foods are called 'complete protein sources'.

'Incomplete protein sources' are any other food sources that provide protein but not all of the essential amino acids, for example, beans, peas and nuts. These food sources must be combined with other food sources that have the missing essential amino acids, so that protein can be made in the body. Some examples of complementary foods are rice eaten with beans, or peanut butter on wholewheat bread.

Another reason to be aware of specific food combinations is to enhance the absorption of the protein consumed, combining the foods to take advantage of the strengths of each. For example, if flour is eaten at breakfast (as a piece of toast, for example), with coffee, and a glass of milk is drunk at lunch, each of the protein sources would be absorbed by the body at a lower potential. But if the bread is consumed with the milk at either meal, the higher protein values of both would be absorbed by the body immediately.

Protein Supplements

Protein supplements are used by some people, particularly weight trainers and athletes, but they may be dangerous. Infants under one year of age, and older people with liver or kidney ailments, often cannot handle the highly concentrated doses of protein in commercially prepared supplements. These supplements may not be good value because they usually do not contain a good balance of the essential amino acids. This is true of those made from non-animal products such as soy.

Six of the essential amino acids are usually present in good quantities in these supplements, but methionine and tryptophan are usually found in lesser amounts. Since 910mg of methionine and 245mg of tryptophan are the recommended daily allowances, check how much of these are contained in a supplement. This is especially important if your diet is lacking in either one or both of these amino acids, and you are relying on the supplement to account for most or all of your protein needs.

A better and cheaper alternative to a supplement is powdered milk. If your diet is deficient in protein, you might consider using egg whites (or egg substitutes), non-fat milk, fish, or chicken. It will be less expensive and have more and higher-quality protein.

The United States Olympic Committee's Center for Sports Nutrition and the British Olympic Association advise against amino acid supplements. They have not been found to be effective and they can cause liver and kidney damage, loss of calcium, dehydration, and a type of arthritis called gout (International Center for Sports Nutrition and the United States Olympic Committee, Sports Medicine Division, *Protein: Implications for athletes,* 1990, pp. 21–22).

FAT

Fat is made of carbon, hydrogen and oxygen. There are nine calories in one gram of fat. In the body, fat is used to develop the myelin sheath that surrounds the nerves. It also aids in the absorption of vitamins A, D, E and K, which are the fat-soluble vitamins. It serves as a protective layer around the vital organs, and it is an insulator against the cold. Fat is also a great concentrated energy source, and, of course, its most redeeming quality is that it adds flavour and juiciness to food!

Types of Fats

There are three major kinds of fats (fatty acids):
1. saturated fats;
2. mono-unsaturated fats;
3. polyunsaturated fats.

The types and amounts of these fats vary from food to food.

Saturated fats are 'saturated' with hydrogen atoms. They are generally solid at room temperature and are most often found in animal fats, egg yolks, and whole milk products. Since these are the fats that are primarily responsible for raising the blood cholesterol level, and hardening the arteries, they should be minimized.

Mono-unsaturated fats (oleic fatty acids) have room for two hydrogen ions to double-bond to one carbon. They are liquid at room temperature and are found in great amounts in olive, peanut, and canola (rapeseed) oils. Dietary mono-unsaturated fats have been shown to have the greatest effect on the reduction of cholesterol, thereby contributing a positive effect in slowing the process of artery-hardening (atherosclerosis).

Polyunsaturated fats (linoleic fatty acids) have at least two carbon double bonds available, which translates into space for at least four hydrogen ions. Polyunsaturated fats are also liquid at room temperature and are found in the highest proportion in vegetable sources. Sunflower, corn, and linseed oils are good sources of this type of fat.

Polyunsaturated fatty acids of the omega-3 type may also contribute to the prevention of atherosclerosis. This information seems to be specific to the consumption of fish rather than fish-oil pills. Fish-oil pills may even raise the blood cholesterol level, so self-prescribing these pills is not advisable. The best fish to consume are cold-water fish such as salmon, trout and herring. In addition, some studies suggest that dietary polyunsaturated fats, when consumed in large amounts, may have a harmful effect, worsening atherosclerosis if they are not also consumed with adequate anti-oxidants (see Chapter 20).

Requirements

The minimum requirement for fat in the diet is considered to be between 10 and 20 per cent of the total calories consumed. The absolute maximum should be 30 per cent. The average consumption in the developed world is still above 30 per cent, but it has been declining since the 1970s. Most people consume between 35 and 50 per cent of their total calories in fats, typically with a high level of saturated fats – the fats that should be avoided.

A high fat intake, especially saturated fats, tends to raise blood cholesterol levels in many people. In order to lower blood cholesterol level, to decrease the chances of developing hardened arteries, a diet low in fat is recommended, with the saturated fat intake at 10 per cent or less of the total diet; additionally, less than 300mg of cholesterol should be consumed daily. Simply, the total calories from fat should be kept at less than one-third of the total intake, and twice as much polyunsaturated and mono-unsaturated fats should be eaten as saturated fats.

Sources of Different Fats

Corn oil or sunflower oil margarines are better than butter in terms of the ratio of polyunsaturated to saturated fats. Butter has 17g of saturated fat to one gram of polyunsaturated fat, while sunflower margarine has one gram of saturated fat to 2.5g of polyunsaturated fat. In order to make margarine stay solid at room temperature, hydrogen gas is bubbled through the oil to saturate the open bonds chemically. This leaves a chemically saturated polyunsaturated fat, called a trans-fatty acid, which is now thought to be harmful.

The harder the margarine, the more it has been through the hydrogenation process, and the more chemically saturated polyunsaturated fats, or trans-fatty acids, there are in the margarine. Eating such a margarine will increase blood trans-fatty acid, and the risks of this are still being explored. While it is known that saturated fat increases blood cholesterol which, in turn, increases the risk of heart disease, the consumption of margarine may also be a risk factor in heart disease due to the trans-fatty acids. Many brands of margarine now contain virtually no trans-fatty acids.

When buying foods, especially biscuits, cookies and crackers, always check the type of fat used. Avoid those with palm kernel oil and coconut oil, and be aware of the hydrogenated oils used. While a hydrogenated safflower or canola oil may still have an acceptable fat ratio, a hydrogenated peanut or cottonseed oil may not contain the desired levels of unsaturated fats.

Eggs, another staple in the average diet, contain a great deal of cholesterol and saturated fat. The American Heart Association suggests that no more than four egg yolks should be eaten per week, including yolks that are hidden in other foods, such as cakes, custards, bread, noodles and waffles. An egg yolk contains nearly 300mg of cholesterol, which is the recommended daily *maximum* for cholesterol intake. In addition, the saturated fat in the yolk contributes to the blood cholesterol profile in a negative way. Egg white is the best source of protein in the diet, but the yolk is the worst source of fat, and something to be avoided.

Low-cholesterol egg substitutes are now available, with the yolk removed and substituted by corn oil, non-fat dry milk, and other substances. This reduces the cholesterol level of one egg to less than one mg, and eliminates all the saturated fat. The egg substitute can also be used in cooking where eggs are required. In baking, it is recommended that you use an egg substitute, or replace one egg with two egg whites and no yolks. Egg substitutes can be found in the frozen food or egg sections at the supermarket.

Whole milk, another diet staple, contains 3½ per cent fat, accounting for nearly half of its total calories (160 per pint). Low-fat milk contains 1–2 per cent fat, and about 130 calories per pint, and skimmed or non-fat milk has minimal, if any, fat. Each type of milk contains the same amount of protein, carbohydrate and calcium, so skimmed or non-fat milk is good as a high-protein, low-calorie, low-fat food.

Cholesterol in the diet is less important than saturated fats in terms of controlling the blood cholesterol level, and saturated fats should, therefore, be greatly reduced. The major sources of saturated fats – red meats, butter, egg yolks, chicken skin, and other animal fats – should be greatly decreased. Keep track of both your total fat intake and your intake of saturated and polyunsaturated fats to become better aware of your potential risk for heart disease. For example, one egg contains 5.6g of fat and only 0.7g of polyunsaturated fat; an equal weight of hamburger contains 8.7g of fat and only 0.4g of polyunsaturated fat.

It may be possible to reverse the arterial fat build-up by changing to a diet that is very low in fat. The combination of a very low-fat diet with aerobic exercise has been shown to reduce the fat that can line the arteries.

CARBOHYDRATES

Carbohydrates are made from carbon, hydrogen, and oxygen, just like fats, but 'carbs' are generally a simpler type of molecule. There are four calories in one gram of carbohydrate. If not used immediately for energy as sugar (glucose), they are either stored in the body as glycogen (the stored form of glucose), or synthesized into fat and stored.

Simple and Complex Carbohydrates

Some carbohydrates cannot be broken down by the body's digestive processes. These are called fibres (*see* below). The digestible carbohydrates are of two types – simple and complex. Simple carbohydrates are the most readily usable energy source in the body and include sugar, honey and fruit. Complex carbohydrates are the starches. They also break down into sugar for energy, but their breakdown is slower than with simple carbs. They also bring with them various vitamins and minerals.

People in developed countries often eat too many simple carbohydrates. These are often called 'empty calories', because they have no vitamins, minerals or fibres. Someone who uses a great deal of energy can consume these empty calories without potential weight gain, but they will cause most people to put on weight. The average person consumes 125lb (55kg) of sugar per year, equivalent to one teaspoon every 40 minutes, night and day. Since each teaspoon of sugar contains 17 calories, this amounts to 231,000 calories or 66lb (30kg) of poten-

tial body fat if this energy is not used as fuel for daily living.

High-carbohydrate diets that are especially high in sugar may be hazardous to the health, increasing the amount of triglycerides produced in the liver. These triglycerides are blood fats that contribute to hardening of the arteries. Aerobic exercise reduces triglycerides. Also, a diet high in simple carbohydrates can lead to obesity, which can then result in the development of late-onset diabetes.

FIBRE

Fibre is that part of plant foods that is not digestible. It helps to move the food through the intestines by increasing their peristaltic (wave-like) action. Vegetable fibres are made up chiefly of cellulose, an indigestible carbohydrate that is the main ingredient in the cell walls of plants. Plant-eating animals, such as cows, can digest cellulose and make it into useable carbohydrates. Meat-eating animals, such as humans, do not have the proper enzymes in their digestive tracts to metabolize cellulose.

Bran (which includes the husks of wheat, oats, rice, rye, and corn) is another type of fibre. It is indigestible because of the silica in the outer husks. Some of the fibres, such as wheat bran, corn, and barley are insoluble. Their major function is to add bulk to the faeces and to speed the digested foods through the intestines. This reduces the risk of constipation, intestinal cancer, appendicitis, and diverticulosis.

Diverticulosis

Diverticulosis is an intestinal problem that is now one of the most common intestinal disorders in Western nations – one person in three over the age of fifty has it to some degree. The *diverticulae* are pouches similar to small hernias in the intestinal wall. They are caused either by a fold of muscle in the interior wall that pushes outwards, or by a weakness in the internal muscle itself. In either case, the pouch may fill with faecal matter and become infected. Experts now believe that these pouches are the final stages of a long-term lack of dietary fibre.

Soluble Fibres

Some types of fibres are soluble; they can be somewhat dissolved in water. Pectin, commonly found in raw fruits (especially apple skins and the rinds of citrus fruits), oat and rice brans, and some gums from the seeds and stems of tropical plants (such as guar and xanthin) are soluble fibres. These fibres can pick up certain substances, such as dietary cholesterol and bile salts, as they move through the intestines. One and a half cups of oat bran cereal can reduce blood cholesterol by up to 7 per cent. These fibres can therefore aid in the reduction of heart disease and intestinal cancers, and they are also believed to reduce the chance of developing gallstones.

Weight Reduction

Foods high in fibre are also valuable in weight-reducing diets because they speed the passage of foods through the digestive tract, thereby cutting the amount of possible absorption time. They also reduce the hunger pangs experienced by a dieter, because they fill the stomach. A large salad with a diet dressing provides very few calories, but enough cellulose to fill the stom-

ach, cut the hunger, and move other foods through the intestinal passage.

Fibre in the Diet

Dietitians urge everyone to include more fibre in their diet. We should be particularly conscious of the benefits of whole-grain cereals, bran, and fibrous vegetables. Root vegetables (carrots, beets and turnips) and leafy vegetables are very good sources of fibre. The average diet has between 10–20g of fibre in it per day. The recommendation is to eat at least 25–35g of fibre per day to reduce the risk of colon cancer.

WATER

Water is called the 'essential non-nutrient', because it provides no nutritional value and yet, without it, the body cannot live. Water makes up approximately 60 per cent of the adult body.

Water is used to cool the body through perspiration, it carries nutrients to and waste products from the cells, it helps cushion the vital organs, and is an essential part of the make-up of all body fluids and cells.

The body has about 18 sq ft of skin (5 sq m) containing about two million sweat glands. On a comfortable day, a person will perspire about half a pint (0.25 litre) of water. Somebody exercising on a severely hot day may lose as much as 14 pints (8 litres) of water; this needs to be replaced, or severe dehydration can result. Ideally, everyone should drink eight glasses (2 litres) of water, or its equivalent in other fluids, a day (although this quantity depends on the climate, the altitude, the type of foods eaten, and the amount of activity).

FURTHER READING

Pennington, Jean, and Church, Helen, *Food Values of Portions Commonly Used* (Harper & Row); lists all foods and their protein (including each amino acid), fat and carbohydrate compositions, plus most vitamins and minerals.

CHAPTER 20
Vitamins and Minerals

VITAMINS

Vitamins are organic compounds that are essential in small amounts for the growth and development of animals and humans. They act as *enzymes* (catalysts) which facilitate many of the body processes. While there is controversy about the importance of consuming excess vitamins, it is acknowledged that a minimum amount of vitamins is needed for proper functioning. Now that the destructive impact of free oxygen radicals (*see* below) has been established, it is generally recommended that certain vitamins be included in the daily intake of these nutrients at a level higher than that recommended earlier.

Water-Soluble and Fat-Soluble Vitamins

Some vitamins are soluble only in water; others need fat to be absorbed by the body. The water-soluble vitamins – B complex and C – are more fragile than the fat-soluble vitamins. This is because they are more easily destroyed by the heat of cooking and, if boiled, they lose a little of their potency into the water. Since they are not stored by the body, they should be included in the daily diet.

The fat-soluble vitamins – A, D, E and K – need oils in the intestines in order to be absorbed by the body. They are more stable than the water-soluble vitamins and are not destroyed by normal cooking methods. Because they are stored in the body, there is the possibility of ingesting too much of them, especially vitamins A and D.

Artificial Supplements

Nutritional researchers disagree as to whether vitamin supplements are necessary. They do, however, generally agree that natural vitamins are exactly the same as synthetically prepared vitamins. Thus, synthetically made ascorbic acid *is* vitamin C, and there is no need to take rose hips or acerola types of the vitamin in order to get enough vitamin C. Nevertheless, health benefits have been shown in large groups of people consuming a diet high in anti-oxidant vitamins such as vitamin C, but not yet in individuals taking artificial supplements.

Free Oxygen Radicals

Free oxygen radicals are single atoms of oxygen that can combine with many molecules and tissues. They are harmful substances produced by many natural body processes. Physical exercise, for all of its benefits, is a producer of free oxygen radicals, as are smoking and air pollution. In fact, the simple processes of normal living, even sleeping, produce some free oxygen radicals.

Free oxygen radicals are also found in the environment. Air and water pollution, any type of smoke, and even dried milk and eggs are some of the environmental sources of these toxins. In animal and human experiments relating to the effect of the anti-oxidant properties of vitamins C and E against air pollution and smoke, it was found that vitamin C is more effective in protecting against nitrogen dioxide, while vitamin E is more effective against ozone's oxidative effects. It should be noted, though, that for maximum protection against the harmful effects of air pollutants, the recommended dietary allowances for both of these vitamins should be increased.

The free oxygen radicals are implicated in many diseases, particularly mouth, throat, skin, stomach, prostate, colon, oesophagus and lung cancers. They are also suspected of being one of the substances that can start the lesions that develop into hardened arteries and heart disease, and of causing cataracts (a hardening and damaging of the lens of the eye), and infertility. They are also linked to about fifty other diseases, including ulcers, asthma, and high blood pressure.

Vitamin A

Vitamin A is necessary for good eyesight as well as skin. During World War II, Denmark began exporting large amounts of butter and supplemented Danish diets with margarine. Many children developed problems with their eyesight, and it was eventually discovered that the necessary vitamin A, which had been available in the butter, was not being provided by the margarine. Vitamin A was added to the margarine and no further problems developed.

It is possible to get too much of the vitamin A that comes from animal sources such as liver, milk and butter. When this happens the liver can enlarge, there can be a loss of appetite or weight, loss of hair, severe bone and joint pain, and cracking lips. This would probably occur only after consuming twenty times the minimum daily requirement over a long period of time.

Beta carotene is the plant source from which our bodies make vitamin A. Beta carotene does not seem to have the toxicity of vitamin A from animal sources. Beta carotene is a powerful anti-oxidant. Along with other anti-oxidants, including vitamins C and E, and the minerals selenium, zinc, and chromium, beta carotene 'donates' electrons to free oxygen radicals, making them less destructive. Once the beta carotene is converted to vitamin A it is no longer an anti-oxidant.

B-Complex Vitamins

The B-complex vitamins include at least fifteen substances; only six have been termed 'essential'. The B vitamins seem to work together, particularly in the nervous, circulatory, and digestive systems. Since they work together, an overdose of some could result in a deficiency in others.

Vitamin B1 *(thiamin)* is used to help to convert sugars (glucose) into an energy source that can be more readily used in the muscles. For this reason, people who are doing aerobic training must make sure that they have sufficient vitamin B. Without the vitamin, a disease called 'beri beri' can develop, which leads to a lack of energy.

There are other theories about the possible positive effects of the vitamin. There is some evidence that thiamin in doses of over 5mg a day may act as an insect repellent, giving the skin an odour that repels some bugs, including mosquitoes.

The primary function of vitamin B2 (riboflavin) is to convert fatty acids and proteins into sugars that can be used for energy. Riboflavin and vitamin B6 *(pyridoxine)* deficiencies may prove to hamper fitness performance, but, if there is no deficiency, there appears to be no additional benefit from further supplementation of the vitamins. With an increase in exercise training, riboflavin stores in the body have been shown to be reduced, so it may be important to increase the intake of riboflavin when embarking on or increasing an existing exercise programme.

Vitamin B3 *(niacin)* is necessary for the breakdown of glucose into energy. It is therefore essential for endurance athletes. It has also been found to inhibit the growth rate of some cancer cells in rats. Pellagra, a niacin-deficiency disease, can lead to the development of symptoms of mental illness, such as hallucinations.

Vitamin B6 has several roles, but its major function is in the development of proteins from amino acids. It may be an important vitamin for those concerned with building muscle tissue.

Vitamin B12 is necessary for the development of red blood cells and for maintaining the fatty sheath which protects the nerves. The diet of the vegan, who consumes no animal products or by-products, is usually deficient in vitamin B12. This is a concern because a vitamin B12 deficiency, in extreme cases, can cause a loss of brain function. In one study, a group of vegans in England suffered irreversible destruction of nerve fibres in the spinal cord after ten to fifteen years, because of a chronic vitamin B12 deficiency.

Folacin (folic acid) is a component of many tissues. If there is not enough of the vitamin present, the work of the cells is impaired. It is now known that it is an essential nutrient for pregnant mothers because a deficiency can cause severe birth defects.

Excessive B vitamins can affect the efficiency of prescription drugs. For example, riboflavin can interfere with the effects of the antibiotic tetracycline. Pyridoxine can interfere with levadopa, which is often prescribed for Parkinson's disease, and folic acid can lessen the effects of an anti-epileptic drug.

Vitamin C

Vitamin C is essential in the production of collagen, which is a protein substance that holds together body tissues, such as bones, teeth, and skin. It is also important for healing wounds. In addition, it helps the body to use iron and assists in the creation of the thyroid hormone thyroxin. It is also a powerful anti-oxidant, and it is probably the most controversial of all the vitamins.

Without 10mg of vitamin C a day, scurvy can develop. In the past, before the effects of vitamin C were known, whole armies were decimated by this disease – it is estimated that over 10,000 seamen died in the early days of exploration, because they didn't have enough vitamin C. Once fresh citrus fruits were added to their diet, scurvy ceased to be a problem.

Vitamin C is made from glucose, a simple sugar found in ordinary table sugar. In order to convert the glucose into vitamin C, a special liver enzyme is required. Most animals have the ability to make this conversion, but humans do not have the correct enzyme in their system, so they must take in vitamin C from an outside source, such as oranges.

Most of the research relating to vitamin C has dealt with whether or not it can cure or prevent the common cold, but most studies have been inconclusive. Since there are at least 113 distinct viruses known to be able to cause a cold, it is unlikely that any one vitamin could work to limit all the viruses. However, it does seem to have some positive effects in protecting against colds. This may be due to the effects of collagen building.

Smokers may require more vitamin C than other people, because of the protective effects of vitamin C as an anti-oxidant. It has been shown that smokers have lower blood levels of vitamin C than non-smokers, and smokers with a vitamin C deficiency have a greater chance of developing certain oral mucosal lesions.

Vitamin D

Vitamin D is seldom found to be deficient in the average diet. It can also be made by the effect of sunlight on a cholesterol near the skin. Just two to three fifteen-minute periods in the sun per week should produce sufficient vitamin D.

Vitamin E

Vitamin E, like vitamin C, has many advocates who claim unproven benefits from its use. Some claim that vitamin E may be able to help cells live longer. This does not mean that vitamin E will slow the ageing process, but it may indicate that the vitamin, because of its anti-oxidant properties, can be a shield to certain environmental stresses, such as smog, radiation, and other pollutants. When cells treated with vitamin E were exposed to such environmental stresses, only 30 per cent stopped reproducing, compared to 90 per cent of the untreated cells.

Another major claim for vitamin E is that it helps the human heart, and has been beneficial in the treatment of animal heart problems. This was first reported at the 1972 American Heart Association meeting. Some research now indicates that effective vitamin E supplementation may reduce heart attacks by as much as 40 per cent. The lower rate of heart disease among those with high vitamin E levels was documented by the World Health Organization, which found that a low level of vitamin E was the most important predictor of heart disease; 62 per cent of those dying had these low levels. Heart pain (angina) and cancers also seem to be reduced by adequate intakes of vitamin E. One factor may be that vitamin E somehow blocks some of the clotting action of vitamin K, so it reduces the blood's tendency to clot.

Vitamin K

Vitamin K is necessary for two of the fourteen steps necessary for the blood to clot. It is found in many foods, and in most people it is produced in the intestines by bacteria.

MINERALS

Minerals are usually structural components of the body, but they sometimes participate in certain body processes. The body uses many minerals – phosphorus, calcium, and magnesium for strong teeth and bones; zinc for growth; chromium for carbohydrate metabolism; and copper and iron for haemoglobin production in the blood. *See also* the appendix for a more detailed analysis of minerals.

Iron

Iron is used primarily in developing haemoglobin, which carries the oxygen in the red blood cells. Women need more iron than men do until they go through menopause (18mg a day), at which time their iron requirements drop to the same as that of men (10mg a day). Iron deficiency, common in women athletes, may impair athletic performance and should be corrected with supplementation.

Magnesium

Magnesium is the eighth most abundant element on the earth's surface. It seems to help activate enzymes essential to energy transfer. It is crucial for effective contraction of the muscles. Exercise depletes this element, so supplementation may be needed. When it is not present in sufficient amounts, twitching, tremors, and undue anxiety may develop.

Calcium

Calcium is primarily responsible for the building of strong bones and teeth. A diet that is chronically low in calcium will obviously have a negative effect on bone strength. The result of this is brittle and porous bones with ageing, a condition known as osteoporosis. This is diagnosed when the bone density shows a loss of 40 per cent of the necessary calcium. It happens quite often in older people, especially women who have gone through menopause or have had their ovaries removed, as oestrogen seems to serve a protective function against bone loss.

The inclusion of adequate calcium (which may be higher than the current RDA or Recommended Daily Allowance) in teenage and young adult years can aid in the development of peak bone mass, which can help prevent osteoporosis later on in life. Another contributing factor to osteoporosis is the imbalance of phosphorus to calcium in the typical diet. Calcium and phosphorus work together, and should be consumed in a 1 to 1 ratio. However, the average diet is much higher in phosphorus than calcium, leading to a leeching of calcium from the bones to make up for this imbalance.

Calcium is also necessary for strong teeth, nerve transmissions, blood clotting, and muscle contractions. Without enough calcium, muscle cramps often result. Skipping milk, with its necessary calcium, may be one of the causes of menstrual cramping for some girls. The uterus is a muscle and muscles need both sodium and calcium for proper contractile functioning.

Fluoride

Fluoride deficiency may be a primary nutritional deficiency in the western world. It is a major preventer of cavities and dental caries, helping to build stronger bones and teeth.

Potassium

Potassium is a chief mineral in cell growth. A deficiency can cause impaired nerve and muscle functions, ranging from paralysis to minor weakness, loss of appetite, nausea, depression, apathy, drowsiness, confusion, heart failure, and even death.

Studies that have shown an increase in blood pressure when sodium intake is high have also shown that blood pressure is decreased when the potassium intake is increased. A 1 to 1 ratio of sodium to potassium is considered good. Most people take in much more sodium than desirable and too little potassium.

Sodium

Sodium, along with potassium, helps to maintain the body's water balance. Too much, in some people, can raise the blood pressure because too much water is retained. Since it is the major mineral ingredient in sweat, it may need to be increased in very hot weather or when an athlete perspires too much.

Trace Minerals

Trace minerals are those that are found in the body in very small amounts. Nearly every element found in the body is 'essential', but the trace minerals are required in small amounts and are generally abundantly found in the diet, so there is little reason for dietary deficiency. Usually foods high in calcium and iron are high in the other necessary trace minerals. The trace minerals include the following:
1. *copper* helps in the production of red blood cells; the metabolism of glucose (sugar), with the release of energy, in the formation of fats in the nerve walls; and the formation of connective tissues; deficiency of copper is very rare;
2. *manganese* is used in fat and carbohydrate metabolism, pancreas development, prevention of bone defects, muscle contraction, and many other functions; it has not yet been observed as a human deficiency;
3. *zinc* is an ingredient in insulin and is used in carbohydrate metabolism; it is necessary for the normal growth of organs, the prevention of anaemia, and the growth of all tissues, and helps in wound healing; zinc in excess of the recommended daily amount interferes with copper absorption and decreases the level of HDL cholesterol (the 'good' cholesterol) in the blood;
4. *chromium* helps to regulate blood sugar and to metabolize fats and carbohydrates; it is also an anti-oxidant;

5. *selenium* helps to form the enzymes that neutralize the free oxygen radicals; because of this, it seems to help prevent cancers.

VITAMIN OR MINERAL SUPPLEMENTS

The ideal measure to take, if you suspect any vitamin or mineral deficiency is to redress or correct your diet. Most people get sufficient amounts of vitamin D without a supplement, but many are very low in magnesium, and most women are low in iron, and may want to include these as a supplement. Anyone who doesn't eat citrus fruits or tomatoes may be low in vitamin C. Those who don't eat meat or wheat may be low in the B vitamins, and those who don't eat wholegrain cereals may be low in vitamin E.

There will be situations in which it may not be possible to make the necessary changes in diet. Those on a weight-reducing diet will find it difficult to get all the vitamins and minerals they need, so it is a good idea for them to take a multivitamin and mineral supplement. It is also difficult to maintain an ideal diet while travelling, and a multivitamin pill may provide an 'insurance policy'.

The National Institute for Aging Research suggests supplements. Their recommendation is 17,000 to 50,000 International Units of beta-carotene, 250 to 1,000mg of vitamin C, and 100 to 400 International Units of vitamin E. These recommendations were the conclusion of a number of experts who studied 200 investigations during the last twenty years (*To take anti-oxidant pills or not? The debate heats up*, Tufts Nutrition Letter, 12:3, May 1994, p. 3).

Labelling is often confusing. If the label states 100mg of magnesium gluconate or

5.4mg of magnesium, or 325mg of calcium lactate or 42 mg of calcium, both mean the same in terms of meeting the body's requirements for magnesium or calcium.

If you purchase supplements, try to match the gaps in your diet to the vitamin pill. You might ask a knowledgeable doctor or a registered dietician to analyse your diet, then get the exact dietary supplement or supplements that you need.

Some vitamins, such as A, B1, and C, are inexpensive to produce in supplements, while others, such as pyridoxine, niacin, pantothenic acid or vitamin E, are expensive; consequently, many inexpensive vitamin preparations have the cheaper vitamins without having the others. Make sure you know what vitamins or minerals you need and in what doses, and check with your doctor that the supplement you've chosen best suits your needs.

Supplementation with vitamin pills containing anti-oxidants above required levels does not appear to increase the body's aerobic capacity; however, a deficiency of vitamin C and/or vitamin E has been shown to decrease endurance capacity. In addition, a high intake of anti-oxidants does not appear to prevent oxidative injury to cells during exercise, but it does appear to help decrease oxidative injury both at rest and after exercise.

CHAPTER 21

Sensible Eating and Supplementation

SENSIBLE EATING

In order to eat sensibly, an athlete needs an understanding of the basic principles of nutrition. The nutrients must appear in the diet in proper quantities, and the calories must be at the right level to maintain the desired weight. Allowing obesity to develop can lead to problems such as diabetes, high blood pressure, and heart disease. Incorrect eating can increase the risk of injuries and illnesses.

Insufficient water or minerals can lead to heat injuries or to muscle cramps; insufficient calcium and trace minerals can lead to osteoporosis and fractures. A lack of protein can be reflected in a loss of muscle mass, while a lack of some nutrients can increase susceptibility to colds and other illnesses.

Calorie needs change according to climate and the amount of activity. In hot weather, more fluids must be taken to replace water lost through perspiration. Fewer calories are needed, because the body does not need to

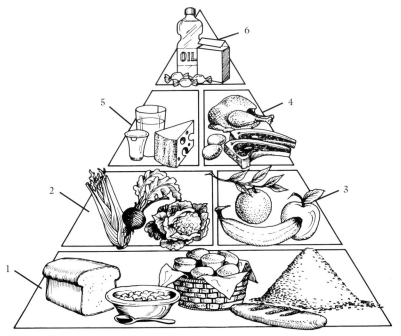

Fig 105. The food pyramid (see opposite).

162

burn as many to maintain its ideal temperature.

An athlete uses a great many calories, and needs more carbohydrates than average. It is, however, not true that an athlete needs much more protein. While caloric needs may be nearly double for an athlete, protein needs are increased only slightly, usually less than 30 per cent. It is not true, either, that athletes require more vitamins and minerals than others do. Giving supplements to athletes who already have a well-balanced diet, with adequate supplementation, has not been shown to improve performance.

THE FOOD GUIDE PYRAMID

The Department of Agriculture of the US Government has devised a suggested diet guide, often called the 'food guide pyramid'. Its base is grain products, followed by fruits and vegetables, then meats and animal products, and, at the top, some fats or sweets, if needed. There are six food groups in the pyramid:

1. grain products (breads, cereals, pastas); recommended servings of 6 to 11 per day;
2. vegetables; 3 to 5 servings per day;
3. fruits; 2 to 4 servings per day;
4. high-protein meats, and meat substitutes (poultry, fish, beans, nuts, eggs); 2 to 3 servings per day;
5. milk products; 2 servings for adults, 3 for children;
6. extra calories, if needed, from fats and/or sweets.

Grain Products

Grain products give the carbohydrates needed for quick energy. A serving size would be one slice of bread, an ounce of dry cereal, or a half-cup of cooked cereal, pasta, or rice. Daily needs are 6 to 11 servings.

The grains are rich in B vitamins, some minerals, and fibre. Whole grains are the best sources of fibres. Refining grains or polishing rice reduces the fibre, the mineral content, and the B vitamins. This occurs in white and wheat bread (not wholewheat), pastas, pastries, and white rice. The flour is often re-fortified with three of the B complex vitamins, but seldom with the other essential nutrients.

To reduce cholesterol levels, and thereby to reduce the chance of developing heart disease, or gall-stones, or to have softer stools, eat more of the soluble fibres (oat bran cereals, wholegrain bread with oats, carrots, potatoes, apples, and citrus juices which contain the pulp of the fruit, or rice bran). To reduce the risk of intestinal cancers, appendicitis, and diverticulosis, eat more insoluble fibres (wholewheat breads and cereals, corn cereals, prunes, beans, peas, nuts, most vegetables, and polished rice).

Vegetables

Vegetables are rich in fibres, beta-carotene, some vitamins and minerals. Among the most nutritious are broccoli, carrots, peas, peppers, and sweet potatoes. For those trying to lose weight, many vegetables are high in water and in fibres, but low in calories. Among these are all greens (lettuce, cabbage, celery), as well as cauliflower. A serving size would be a half-cup of raw or cooked vegetables, or a cup of raw leafy vegetables, and daily needs are 3 to 5 servings.

Fruits

Fruits are generally high in vitamin C and fibre, and relatively low in calories. A serving size would be one-quarter of a cup of dried fruit, half a cup of cooked fruit, three-quarters of a cup of fruit juice, a whole piece of fruit, or a wedge of a melon. You should have 2 to 4 servings daily.

Protein Sources

Protein sources such as meat, eggs, nuts and beans are also high in minerals and vitamins B_6 and B_{12}. A serving would be 2½oz of cooked meat, poultry or fish, 2 egg whites, 4 tablespoons of peanut butter, or one cup and a quarter of cooked beans. The hidden eggs in cakes and biscuits also count. You need 2 to 3 servings a day.

The best meat products to eat are fish, because of the omega 3 oils that reduce blood clotting, egg whites, and poultry without the skin. (Taking the skin off poultry reduces the amount of fat and cholesterol that will be consumed, because much of the fat is carried next to the skin.) Red meat not only has a relatively low quality of protein (after egg white, milk, fish, poultry, and organ meats), but is linked both to cancers (two and a half times the risk for colon cancer), and heart disease. It also carries a large amount of fat, even if the fat on the outside is trimmed off. There is also a great deal of cholesterol in the meat and fat of all land animals.

Fish has a higher quality of protein than meat or poultry, and contains the helpful omega 3 oils, into which they convert the polyunsaturated linolenic fatty acid from plants that they eat. Omega 3 oils interfere with the production of the prostaglandin thromboxane, and therefore help to prevent heart disease by reducing cholesterol, and by making the blood less likely to clot in the arteries.

Milk and Milk Products

Milk and milk products (cheeses, yogurt, ice cream) are high in calcium and protein, as well as some minerals (potassium and zinc), and riboflavin. A serving would be one cup of milk or yogurt, 1½oz of cheese, 2 cups of cottage cheese, 1½ cups of ice cream, or 1 cup of pudding or custard. Adults need 2 servings daily, and children need 3.

Fats and Sweets

Fats and sweets are at the top of the pyramid of foods, and are only there in case a person needs extra calories. Fats should not make up more than 10 to 20 per cent of the diet, preferably in the form of mono-unsaturated and polyunsaturated fatty acids.

Sweets may assist in the development of tooth decay, but are not otherwise harmful if calories are not a problem.

In addition, the following should be noted:

- Avoid milk fat by drinking non-fat milk and milk products, eating frozen desserts made without milk fat, and eating non- or low-fat cheese. Milk is mostly water. The fats in milk are highly saturated – the worst kind – yet the protein quality of milk is second only to that of egg whites.
- Egg yolk contains a great deal of cholesterol and saturated fat, but egg white has the highest rating for protein quality. Make omelettes, or bake, using two egg whites in place of one whole egg.

- Reduce salt; it increases high blood pressure in many people.
- Reduce sugars; they give 'empty' calories, without other nutrients such as vitamins or fibres.
- Reduce fats to between 10 and 20 per cent of your total calories. Use fat-free salad dressing, or vinegar or lemon juice only. Buy a tasty wholegrain bread, and eat it without butter or margarine, or use olive oil, or olive oil and garlic. If calories are not a concern, use a jelly or jam. Avoid frying foods in oil. If you must have oil, use canola (rapeseed), olive, or sunflower oil. Stay away from all fried foods, including potato chips. Fried foods add calories and saturated fats, and increase the chance of intestinal cancers.

BEVERAGES

Beverages make up a large part of every diet. Michael Jacobson, co-director of the Center for Science in the Public Interest in the USA, has assessed them for nutritional value. Rating each drink according to the amount of fat and sugar (higher content = lower rating), and the amount of protein, vitamins, and minerals (higher content = higher rating), his results were as follows:

- skimmed or non-fat milk +47;
- whole milk +38 (lower, because of its fat content);
- orange juice +33;
- Hi-C +4;
- coffee 0;
- coffee with cream –1;
- coffee with sugar –12;
- Kool-Aid –55;
- soft drinks –92.

Milk

Non-fat milk is the best drink for most people. Children should have three to four cups each day, and adults should drink two cups. This requirement can be satisfied by other dairy products – two cups of milk are equivalent to three cups of cottage cheese, or five large scoops of ice cream. In addition to its nutrient value as a developer of bones and organs, milk has been found to help people go to sleep more quickly, and then to sleep longer and more soundly. This may be because of the high content of the amino acid tryptophan, which makes serotonin, the neurotransmitter associated with relaxation.

Calcium in milk is also used in the blood and a deficiency may lead to muscle cramps when exercising. Calcium reduces the chance of developing osteoporosis, and is also needed when a broken bone is mending.

Coffee

Coffee contains several ingredients that may be harmful – stimulants such as caffeine and the xanthines; oils that seem to stimulate the secretion of excess acid in the stomach; and diuretics that eliminate water and some nutrients, such as calcium, from the body. Even two cups a day may increase the risk of bone fractures. (People who drink more coffee usually drink little or no milk.)

Caffeine is found in coffee, tea, and cola drinks. Brewed coffee contains 100–150mg of caffeine per cup, instant coffee about 90mg/cup, tea between 45 and 75mg/cup, and cola drinks from 40 to 60mg/cup. Decaffeinated coffee is virtually free of caffeine, as it contains only 2 to 4mg per cup. The therapeutic dose of caffeine given to people who have overdosed on barbiturates is 43mg. Four strong cups of coffee (600mg), or less if other caffeine-containing drinks are consumed, is enough in some individuals to push the concentration of caffeine in their urine over the limit (12 micrograms per ml) set by the IOC for Olympic competitors.

Caffeine is a central nervous system stimulant. It constricts the blood vessels and elevates the blood pressure. It can also produce the symptoms found in someone suffering from psychological anxiety, including nervousness, irritability, occasional muscle twitching, sensory disturbances, diarrhoea, insomnia, irregular heartbeat, a drop in blood pressure and, occasionally, failures of the blood circulation system.

The oils in coffee irritate the lining of the stomach and the upper intestines, and drinking two or more cups of coffee per day increases the chance of getting ulcers by 72 per cent. Both ordinary and decaffeinated coffee increases the acid secretions in the stomach. Some ingredient other than caffeine is thought to be responsible for increasing stomach acid levels.

Tea

Tea is not as irritating as coffee, but it does contain some caffeine and tannic acid, which can irritate the stomach. Large amounts of tea should be drunk either with milk, to neutralize the acid, or ice to dilute it. Green tea, commonly drunk in the Orient, contains polyphenols, anti-oxidants that may reduce cancer incidence. The black tea commonly drunk in Europe and the USA has fewer of these protective substances. Not much is known about the effects of herbal teas.

Alcohol

There are seven calories in one gram of alcohol, containing no nutritional elements. Alcoholic drinks contribute to the weight problems of many people. People who eat a balanced diet, but also drink alcohol will probably consume too many calories. Cutting down on eating, but still drinking, they may avoid a weight problem, but will probably develop nutritional deficiencies that can result in severe illness. Alcohol is also a central nervous system depressant, which causes a decrease in the metabolism.

The normal dangers of alcohol are the development of alcoholism and the destruction of brain cells, but there are other considerations. Beer or ale, because of its carbonation, affects stomach acid. Gin contains juniper berries and other substances that are stomach and intestinal irritants. While beer may quench the thirst during or after exercise, the alcohol acts as a diuretic so that more water is lost in the urine than is drunk in the beer. Only when the beer is diluted by at least 50 per cent does it start to replace more fluids than it causes to be lost.

Studies have indicated that moderate alcohol consumption (less than three drinks a day) may increase the protective HDL type of blood cholesterol; this effect lasts about twenty-four hours, so little and often is the most healthy way to consume alcohol. Binge drinking has no protective effect on the heart and very obvious negative effects on health and athletic performance. There also seems to be a protective effect from a substance called reservatrol, found in the seeds and skins of grapes. For that reason, red wine may have more protective qualities than other alcoholic drinks, but reservatrol can also be found in grape juice and in grapes, so there is no need to drink the wine to get the benefits.

EATING AND OVER-EATING

We eat to nourish our bodies, but in Europe and the USA many people also eat to reduce stress. Filling our stomach can make us feel totally satisfied in at least one part of our life. When eating to relieve stress, we will probably take in more calories than we need for living. And stress eating is also often done with junk foods – chocolate, ice cream and potato chips are doubly satisfying, because they taste so good while they fill us up.

GAINING WEIGHT

Someone focused on weight gain wants to increase his or her lean body weight – to increase the weight by increasing muscle mass, not fat. The best way to gain weight in muscle is to do resistance-type exercise, such as weight training. (*See* Chapter 22.) Enough protein must be eaten in order to give the body the building blocks it needs to make more muscle. Additionally, B vitamins will be needed, because they help to break down consumed protein into the amino acids necessary to building the body's own protein.

LOSING WEIGHT

Losing weight is a goal for many people, whether to look better, to exercise more efficiently, or to avoid disease. There are a number of ways to determine if you need to.

Those who are over-fat can develop many problems, including: osteoarthritis (from excessive wearing of the joints due to the continual carrying of excess weight), *diabetes mellitus* (from excessive blood sugar), high blood pressure, and hardening of the arter-

ies; so they will probably also die earlier. Over-fat people tend to develop diabetes earlier, form kidney and heart problems sooner, and have less resistance to infection than people of a healthy weight.

If you need to lose weight in order to be a more effective competitor, be careful not to become compulsive; this can lead to anorexia or bulimia. Be sensible about weight loss, and your weight loss programme.

How to Lose Weight

First, find out why you are overweight. If it is genetic, medical help may be needed. If you eat because of stress, find another method to relieve that stress, such as exercise or relaxation techniques (see Chapter 16). If you over-eat because you must have something in your mouth, try gum or a low-calorie food. If your problem is a lack of exercise, start an effective exercise programme. If you simply consume too many calories, change your diet.

To start a weight loss programme, you need to be willing to make permanent lifestyle changes. The majority of dieters cannot make such a commitment; that is why 95 per cent of dieters have regained all of their lost weight within five years, 40 per cent of women and 25 per cent of men are on a diet at any one time. The average American goes on 2.3 diets a year. The average diet is not successful. A pattern of continually gaining and losing is frustrating, so you will have to determine whether you honestly want a healthier lifestyle. A proper lifestyle change to healthy eating and effective exercise will pay many mental, physical, and social dividends.

Reducing Body Fat

Most of our body fat comes from fat that we eat, but each type of food requires energy to digest it. More energy is needed to digest carbohydrates than fat. For example, from 25g of carbohydrate, yielding 100 calories, 23 per cent of the calories will be used to convert the carbohydrate to body fat. Fats are converted into body fat using less energy; 11g of fat represents 99 calories, but it only takes 3 per cent of those calories to convert it, and 96 calories of body fat can be deposited. Approximately 100g of carbohydrate consumed in the diet, if not used for energy, will become 8.5g of body fat, while approximately 100g of fat from the diet will become 10.75g of body fat.

To lose one pound of fat per week, you must have a net deficit of 500 calories per day. (One pound of fat contains 3,500 calories.) This may be done solely by decreasing your food intake by 500 calories per day, but your metabolism will slow down over time to allow for the decrease in food energy, and it will be harder and harder to continue to lose fat.

Similarly, you could choose to increase your activity level to burn off 500 calories a day, but it would take a great deal of energy to achieve this, and it could be dangerous if you are not currently exercising.

Calorie-Counting and Exercise

The best method is to combine calorie reduction with exercise to achieve your goal. Aerobic exercise will keep your metabolism up as you lose the fat, and you won't have to restrict your calories to an impossible extreme, because you will be burning off energy each time you exercise.

Calories are used both during and after exercise. The longer and more vigorous the exercise, the more the metabolism is increased, and the longer after the exercise is completed will the calorie expenditure be increased over normal.

Reasonable amounts of exercise will not make you eat more. In fact, exercising just before a meal can dull your appetite, and decrease your desire for calories.

AN EFFECTIVE DIET FOR ATHLETES

Eating the right nutrients in sufficient quantities is absolutely fundamental to increasing athletic potential, reducing the likelihood of injuries, and rehabilitating injuries after they occur. The body cannot make the necessary tissues or expend the required energy without the right nutrients in the right proportions. Serious attention is required in this area of training, both for the recreational sportsperson, and for the competing athlete.

Muscle, blood or bone cannot be built without protein and minerals. Carbohydrates stored in the liver, and adequate water and carbohydrate replacement are essential for an endurance athlete. Carbohydrate replacement in the muscles is also essential for quick recovery from exercise. Enough calcium is needed in the diet in order to prevent bone injuries. Sufficient vitamin C is important for quick recovery.

SUPPLEMENTATION FOR ATHLETES

Supplements claiming to improve performance, prevent fatigue, or prolong life have no proven benefit, but can be used as an insurance policy if there is a risk of inadequate diet. This supplementation is generally specific. They can affect an athlete's chance of injury by increasing the risk, as steroids do, or decreasing the risk, by ensuring adequate fluid intake during and after exercise.

BUILDING MUSCLE

Building muscle requires hard work, especially with resistance exercises. It is more effective if the diet has sufficient amounts of high-quality protein. Protein pills are a waste of money. Egg whites, skimmed or powdered milk, fish or chicken have more and better protein for less money. Certain vitamins and minerals are also essential in building muscle tissue (*see* Chapter 20).

STEROIDS

Androgenic steroids are legitimately given to people who have a medical need for more testosterone, because they do not secrete enough of the hormone naturally, or to children who are growth hormone-deficient. Steroids have been used illicitly for many years by body-builders and athletes for whom strength is a major concern; they generally take the drugs at a much higher dose than those who have a medical need.

Various steroids, while generally stimulating muscle growth for those who are working with heavy resistance exercises, may have a negative effect, which may vary from drug to drug. Men may experience brittle bones that frequently break, high blood pressure, breast tenderness, liver damage, sperm count reduction, a reduction in the size of the testicles, and occasionally death. Women can develop the same problems as men, and may also encounter male pattern baldness, a

deeper voice, and enlargement of the clitoris.

Teenage boys may take drugs to develop a body that they think is more attractive to girls. It may speed up their secondary sex characteristic development, but it may also make their bones harden too early, and then stunt their growth.

The negative effects of anabolic steroids far outweigh any benefits. That is why they are outlawed.

ERGOGENIC AIDS FOR ENDURANCE

The oxygen-carrying capacity of the blood, the aerobic capacity, can best be increased by doing endurance exercise (running, swimming, or cycling) for long distances. If there are sufficient amounts of protein, iron, copper, and B vitamins, more red blood cells will be developed, so that each unit of blood will have more oxygen-carrying capacity. This will allow the oxygen breathed into the lungs to get more effectively to the tissues where it is needed.

Illegal methods of achieving this same goal are blood doping (injecting blood, usually the athlete's own, back into the athlete), and the injection of erythropoietin (EPO, a red blood cell producer). While EPO is found naturally in the body, injecting it to get an even higher effect is unethical, and may thicken the blood so much that a stroke or a heart attack occurs.

A legal method of getting more red blood cells is to live at a higher altitude. It was once thought that both living and exercising at higher altitude was effective, but it is now known that living at high altitude but exercising at a lower altitude is more effective.

CARBOHYDRATES

Carbohydrate Loading

Increasing carbohydrate fuel for endurance events can be done by carbohydrate loading before a long-distance race, or a game requiring endurance. It can be done during the event.

Carbohydrate loading before an event can be done by reducing carbohydrates to about 50 per cent of the diet for three days, then increasing them to 70 per cent of the calories for the last three days. Some people have used an even more extreme approach by reducing carbohydrates to under 40 per cent for the first three days, and increasing to 80 to 90 per cent for the last three days. This extreme regime can have some negative consequences, so is generally not recommended.

Carbohydrate Replacement

Carbohydrate replacement during an event has been found greatly to increase endurance. Maltodextrin (glucose polymer) has been shown to be more effective than a simple sugar drink, and both are far better than water for carbohydrate replacement. If you want to use a carbohydrate replacement drink for prolonged endurance exercise, be certain that the ingredient list includes maltodextrin or glucose polymers.

Immediate replacement of the carbohydrates lost during exercise can shorten the recovery period after a workout or a competition. Maximum recovery from a weight-training session, or an endurance activity such as running, cycling or swimming, cannot happen without it. Many weight-trainers think that they need protein replacement, but in fact they need carbohydrates.

Fluids

Fluid replacement is essential for people who are sweating either because of exercise or the outside temperature. The fluid can be replaced at the same time as carbohydrates are replaced with a glucose polymer drink. Other popular drinks include dextrose or another sugar, along with some of the minerals that are lost in perspiration. Sodium chloride (salt), magnesium, potassium and calcium are among the common additives to such drinks.

Several minerals are lost in initial sweat, but with time, the sweat becomes nearly pure water. If energy replacement is not the objective, and cost is a problem, just drink lots of water. It may take slightly longer to be absorbed than the salt/sugar solution (in most sports drinks), but will do the job effectively. Sportspeople generally do not take in as much water as they lose during exercise, and should therefore 'force feed' themselves more water.

INCREASING ANAEROBIC CAPACITY

Creatine

Increasing anaerobic (that is, without the oxygen which is breathed in) capacity can be done legally. Lifting a weight, beginning a running or swimming sprint, a jump or vault, a golf swing, a tennis serve, the short sprints necessary while playing basketball, soccer, hockey and other such sports, are all short anaerobic bursts of energy. The ability to develop short-term bursts of energy can be improved by the administration of creatine.

Creatine is a naturally occurring compound made in the body, primarily in the liver, but also in the kidneys and the pancreas. It is essential for muscle functioning. It is found in good amounts in both meat and fish, but some of it is destroyed in cooking. A normal diet provides about one gram a day. Some athletes, particularly in events that require repetitive surges of power, supplement with this natural body substance. It is not banned by the Olympic Committee. Not everyone benefits because there is a maximum concentration of creatine that can be held in the muscle (60 millimolar), and they may already have that. Also, one of the immediate effects of supplementation is to cause fluid retention in the muscles; the athlete may immediately put on 5lb (2kg) or more in weight.

ATP

A number of chemical actions supply energy to the individual muscle fibre. The primary energy source is called ATP (adenosine triphosphate), used for energy in all cells. As the name implies, there are three ('tri') phosphates in the molecule. Energy is released when one of these phosphates is broken off. This energy supplies the power for the muscle fibre to draw up on itself (to contract). There is enough ATP in the muscle to last for almost a second. If it is not re-synthesized there will be no more fuel for the muscle.

The ATP is re-synthesized by taking the phosphate in creatine phosphate that is also present in the cell. But just as the ATP storage in the cell will last for only about a second, the creatine phosphate available will last for only about five seconds. The use of these substances for energy is called anaerobic.

In order to continue to supply the muscles with an energy source, the cells use the food (carbohydrates, proteins, and fats) without oxygen (anaerobic) for up to 20 seconds. From a few seconds onwards the food is progressively used with oxygen that is in the blood and is continuously being breathed in. The muscle fibres are now being fuelled aerobically.

Creatine Supplementation

Anaerobic work is short term, and supplementation with creatine monohydrate has been found useful to increase the speed of recovery of the muscles that work anaerobically. After the fifth or more effort a few seconds apart, the subsequent sprints are better than they would have been without supplementation.

Experiments have used a loading dose of 5g of creatine monohydrate four times a day for five days, then 2g a day. (Taking more will not help, as the tissues can only hold a certain amount, and the excess will be excreted in the urine.) It has also been shown that 2g per day will raise muscle creatine to its maximum level after four weeks, and this dose is much closer to the normal dietary intake.

(We are indebted to Dr Anna Casey of the Department of Physiology and Pharmacology of the Faculty of Medicine and Health Sciences at the Queen's Medical Centre of Nottingham, England, for her important research in the area of creatine supplementation.)

STIMULANTS

Stimulants can increase alertness, strength and endurance. The only legal stimulant available is caffeine. It seems to increase strength by allowing more muscle fibres to be used in a single contraction, and to help endurance by increasing the amount of fuel available to the muscles. It does this by allowing the use of the triglyceride blood fats for energy, thereby saving the muscle sugars (glycogen) for later. Amphetamines and ephedrine were common stimulants, but have been outlawed by the athletic community.

CALORIE USE IN SPORTS

Approximate number of calories used in one hour:

Soccer	450
Cross country skiing at 5 mph (8km/h)	600
Running at 7 mph (11km/h)	670
Running at 9 mph (14.5km/h)	900
Bicycling at 5½ mph (9km/h)	250

Prohibited Classes of Substances and Prohibited Methods

1. Prohibited Classes of Substances

a. Stimulants
b. Narcotics
c. Anabolic Agents
d. Diuretics
e. Peptide and glycoprotein hormones and analogues

2. Prohibited Methods

a. Blood Doping
b. Pharmacological, chemical and physical manipulation

3. Classes of Drugs subject to Certain Restrictions

a. Alcohol
b. Marijuana
c. Local anaesthetics
d. Corticosteroids
e. Beta-blockers

4. Examples of Prohibited Substances*

Amphetamines
Caffeine (more than 12 micrograms per millilitre of urine)
Choronic Gonadotrophin (HCG - human chrorionic gonadotrophin)
Corticotrophin (ACTH)
Dehydroepiandrosterone (DHEA)
Diamorphine (heroine)
Ephedrines
Erythropoietin
Growth Hormone (hGH, somatorophin)
Methadone
Morphine
Testosterone (more than 6 times the normal amount in a competitor's urine)
For a complete list of banned substances contact the British Olympic Association.

Fig 106

CHAPTER 22
Conditioning

Proper conditioning requires a combination of strength, endurance (cardio-vascular or aerobic), flexibility, and power (strength and speed combined), along with whatever co-ordination is needed for your favourite sport. A gymnast needs strength, power and flexibility with some endurance. A marathon runner needs endurance with some flexibility, but not much strength or power. A soccer player needs endurance, power for kicking and sprinting, and flexibility.

Correct conditioning is necessary for performing at your best, and is also important in terms of reducing injuries. Strength training not only makes the muscles stronger but also the bones, countering the effects of osteoporosis. Endurance training not only makes your heart, blood, and lungs more efficient, and increases the immune factors that fight diseases, from colds to cancers, but can also help to reduce the blood fats that can bring on heart disease and stroke. Flexibility exercise makes the body more able, and can eliminate lower-back pain that is so common as we grow older.

Many people exercise for the health benefits (avoiding disease, slowing the ageing process, controlling body weight), and for this they need the endurance or aerobic exercise. Some people exercise to make their body more appealing; this will involve more strength and body-contouring work. However, a great number of people exercise simply to experience the joy of sport.

This group is more likely to experience injuries.

THE PRINCIPLE OF SPECIFICITY

Sports training must be specific to achieve the expected or required outcome – strength, speed, endurance, power, flexibility, or injury prevention. For example, a bench press is absolutely essential if you are a power lifter, and it certainly helps if you use a push-away action in your sport, as in wrestling, American football, putting the shot or boxing. It would help in throwing sports, such as team handball or baseball, but its effectiveness is less and less apparent if you are a swimmer, sprinter, tennis player, or long-distance runner.

To make the best use of workout time, select activities that will aid you the most in preventing injuries and increasing performance. A sportsperson who sprints, such as a soccer player, should include exercise that stretches the hamstrings and buttocks (gluteals), and then contracts them under pressure. Long-distance swimming will not much help the soccer player, who would do better to run. A golfer, or someone who throws in sport, should do exercises which strengthen the rotator cuff muscles in the shoulder. Straight arm pull-downs on a 'lat' machine will greatly increase a swimmer's speed in the water, but doing extra flexibility exercises as a warm-up will actually reduce swimming speed.

Research on the effectiveness of stretching and flexibility work is now being carried on in a number of universities. Australian Dr Greg Wilson, a former world-class power lifter, has the view that the typical strength training used by athletes has been designed primarily by former power lifters, Olympic weight lifters, and body-builders. The exercises they recommend may have worked for them in their sport, but will not necessarily work for swimmers, soccer players, or runners, and may even cause injuries to these athletes, whose lifting technique is often faulty. His views validate the work of one of this book's authors who has long trained Olympic coaches and athletes in the specificity of strength gains.

CARDIO-RESPIRATORY ENDURANCE

If you can run, swim, bicycle, or ski cross-country every day – great! As your body exercises aerobically (using oxygen that you have inhaled since you started the exercise), you begin to get positive changes in your blood. This begins about 40 seconds after you begin to exercise. (Before this, your body is using anaerobic energy and oxygen that is stored in the muscles or circulating in the blood.)

Red Blood Cells

At the aerobic level, several changes begin to occur. More red blood cells are activated. They carry oxygen from the lungs to the muscles, then carbon dioxide is carried from the muscles to the lungs, to be exhaled. While much of the blood is already circulating, the demands of exercise cause blood from other organs, such as the liver and spleen, to flow into the circulatory system.

After exercise, many of these red cells will remain in circulation. In a few days, a large number will go back to storage organs, but if endurance exercise is done daily most of the red cells will keep circulating. The body will recognize that it needs more red cells, so it will create more – as long as it has sufficient protein, iron, copper, vitamin B_{12}, and the other necessary ingredients for new red blood cells.

Fuel is provided to the muscles as follows:
1. oxygen is breathed in from the air, and attracted to the blood cells by the haemoglobin;
2. simple sugars, the simplest usable form of consumed food, are added to the blood;
3. from the atoms in these substances, the body's own energy sources are rebuilt;
4. carbon dioxide and water remain; the carbon dioxide is then exhaled.

A high number of red cells means that the body is more efficient at transporting oxygen to the muscles and carbon dioxide away from them. This is even more important at higher altitudes, where the pressure of oxygen is less.

IMPROVING ENDURANCE

To improve endurance, the heart rate must be significantly increased for at least twenty to thirty minutes. This will give the necessary benefits to reduce heart attack risk. It is wise to work out at least three days a week, and six is better.

The generally accepted standard for endurance training for the fit individual is to exercise until the heart reaches an acceptable level for twenty to thirty minutes. That 'acceptable' level is 60 to 85 per cent of the maximum heart rate – 220 heartbeats per minute, minus your age. So, for a 20-year-old, it would be 200, and he or she should work out with a pulse rate of between 130 and 170, for twenty to thirty minutes. A 40-year-old should work out with a pulse rate of between 117 and 153, and so on. Working at 85 per cent of the maximum heart rate is most desirable, because the heart will be working harder.

Pulse Rates

An average resting pulse rate will be in the 70s, and will drop as a person becomes fitter and fitter. With more red blood cells, and a bigger blood volume filling the heart more efficiently, the heart doesn't have to beat as often to get its work done. A resting pulse rate in the mid-60s reflects a better than average condition, a rate in the 40s shows a body in great shape, and a few world-class endurance athletes have a pulse rate in the 30s.

To check your pulse, put your fingers, not your thumb, on the opposite wrist just above the thumb, or put them a few inches below your ear on the inside of the muscle on the side of your neck. Some people just like to put a hand over the heart and feel the beat. Count for a minute to get your pulse rate, or count for fifteen seconds and multiply by four. If you are exercising, it is often easier to count the beats for only six

seconds, then multiply by ten to get your pulse rate.

AN AEROBIC EXERCISE PROGRAMME

Consult Your Doctor

Before you start an exercise programme, consult your doctor, especially if you haven't exercised routinely for some time, or if you suffer from any medical condition. Get your blood pressure checked, and discuss a sensible exercise regime with the doctor, taking into account your history and state of health.

How to Exercise

Any exercise – cross-country skiing, swimming, running, cycling, sex – that gets your heart beating fast enough to get into your target zone is good. Whatever exercise you are doing, get to your target heart rate and stay there for at least twenty minutes; thirty minutes is better. Warm up before you hit your target range – perform your activity at a slightly slower pace for a few minutes before speeding up to hit your target rate.

At the end of your exercise, cool down by slowing your exercise and letting your heart rate drop. Then finish with some stretching. Some people like to stretch before their aerobic workout – do some aerobic warm-up, such as jogging or skiing, then stretch. Next get into your real aerobic workout, then stretch again after your workout. Stretching after a workout is more important than stretching before, because the connective tissues are more easily and effectively stretched when they are warm.

VO₂ Max Tests

To find out your aerobic condition, have a VO₂ Max test, to measure the maximum amount of oxygen, in millilitres, used per minute per kilo of body weight. The average person generally uses 30 to 40 ml/min/kg (millilitres per minute per kilogram). People who exercise a little by walking or doing leisurely cycling may be in the 40 to 50 range, while top endurance athletes are more likely to be in the 70 to 80 area. Top-level cyclist Miguel Indurain uses 94 ml/min/kg and Bjorn Daehle, the world champion cross-country skier, has measured 95. Most of the top male cross-country skiers are over 90, while the top women cross-country skiers generally measure around 70 to 75 ml/min/kg.

MUSCULAR ENDURANCE

Specific Exercise

An effective aerobic programme is necessary if you want to develop your general level of fitness, reduce your heart attack risk, and increase the effectiveness of your immune system. If you want to improve in your sport, you need specific endurance exercise to develop the muscles you need. Running, walking, swimming, cycling and cross-country skiing will all help keep your heart healthy and improve your level of red blood cells, but your individual muscles also have to have specific endurance.

Using muscles in an endurance activity will develop a better capacity to use the oxygen and sugars that the blood brings to them. There will be more haemoglobin in the muscles, more readily available fuel, and a different type of muscle tissue may even be developed. The arteries that supply blood to the exercising muscles also become larger. This allows for more blood to be brought to the exercising muscle.

Only the muscles that are used in your exercise programme are able to gain these specific benefits, which give them more stamina. A tennis player's playing arm will be in much better condition than the other arm. A swimmer's upper back, chest and arms will show such gains, as will a runner's legs.

Muscle Fibre

There are three different types of muscle fibre, the slow twitch (red or Type I), the intermediate (Type IIa), and the fast twitch (white or Type IIb). The fast twitch fibres contract quickly but cannot do it for many repetitions. Olympic weight-lifters have a high percentage of these because they need one powerful contraction, then rest for many minutes. Endurance athletes have a large percentage of slow twitch fibres; cross-country skiers may have 70 to 80 per cent, while distance runners are likely to have over 80 per cent. These fibres contain more fuel and can contract many times before they are exhausted.

The proportion of each fibre type is genetically inherited, but research indicates that certain training can change this to a small extent. Intermediate fibres may change more towards the fast or the slow twitch type of fibre.

INCREASING STRENGTH

Muscular endurance and muscular strength are very different. Strength is the amount of force generated in one muscular contraction, while endurance is how long muscular contractions can be continued with relatively little resistance. A long-distance runner never needs the maximum force an Olympic weight-lifter needs, but there may be times when more than the normal amount of force is needed, for example, when running up a hill.

Strength is determined primarily by how many individual muscle fibres you can have contracting in one contraction. No one can contract all of the muscle fibres in a muscle at the same time, and few people can contract even 50 per cent of their muscle fibres at one time. Strength training is designed to teach the brain to be able to contract more muscle fibres at one time. As strength is gained in the muscles, the cross-sectional area of the muscle increases so that each fibre can exert a greater force in a contraction. Strength comes from both the nervous system and from the muscles.

STRENGTH EXERCISES

The following exercises will help to condition the muscles. To develop strength, exhaust the muscles in under ten repetitions, preferably in one to three repetitions. If you are working on developing muscular endurance, such as you would use in running a marathon or cycling, do as many repetitions as possible – 25 to 100 would be the right range for most people. The muscles should be exhausted when you finish. It is only by getting your muscles very tired that you will get the best results.

The following exercises will condition you better for sports and reduce your chance of injury:

Abdominal Curl-Up

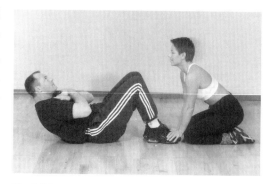

Fig 107

The abdominal muscles are used in every type of exercise; the latest techniques make the exercise more effective:

1. lie on the floor, or on a bed;
2. put your hands on your chest (to avoid pulling on the neck muscles);
3. bring your feet up as close to your hips as possible (so that you don't use the small hip-flexing muscles which attach to the lower back – especially important for women);
4. look at the ceiling and continue looking at the same spot during the exercise (so that you don't stretch the muscles in the back of your neck);
5. raise your shoulders and concentrate on bringing the lower part of your ribs closer to the top of your hips;

6. do as many repetitions as you can, to develop muscular endurance in these muscles.

There are four sets of muscles in the abdominal wall. The *rectus abdominis* does most of the work in the sit-up. Two sets of angled muscles called the 'obliques' also assist in the sit-up, but also work in twisting and sideways bending actions. These exercises work on the obliques.

Twisting Abdominal Curl-Ups

1. Proceed as for the abdominal curl-up;
2. as you raise your shoulders, bring your right shoulder towards your left knee on one repetition, then your left shoulder to your right knee on the next one.

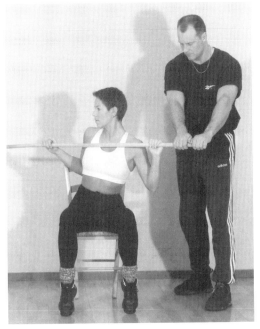

Fig 110

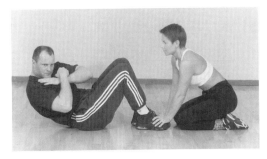

Fig 108

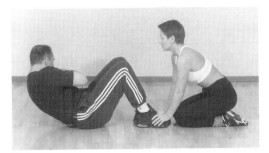

Fig 109

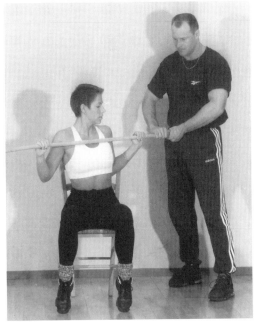

Fig 111

There may be a rotary abdominal machine at your gym, which can be more effective than the twisting sit-up. Alternatively, work with a partner. Sit in a chair holding a rod or broom across your upper chest, and have your partner give resistance to one end of the rod while you twist against it.

Side Sit-Ups

The side sit-up can also develop the abdominal obliques:

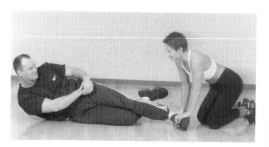

Fig 112

1. put your feet under a sofa or have someone hold them down;
2. while on your side, bring your shoulders and torso upwards.

Leg-Overs

To do leg-overs:

1. while lying on your back, raise your legs so that they are straight over your hips;
2. let them move slowly to the right until they touch the floor;
3. lift them back to the original position, then let them move to the floor to the left.

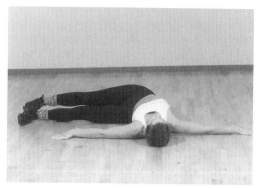

Fig 113

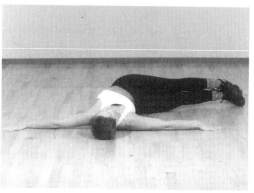

Fig 114

Shoulder Extension

This is an important exercise for swimmers and gymnasts. The upper back muscles (*latissimus dorsi*) and the back of the arm muscles (triceps) are also used in throwing, and for serving and hitting the backhand in tennis. If you belong to a gym, use a pull-down pulley; pull it down with your arms straight.

Alternatively, use stretching bands from a sporting goods store or about 8 to 10ft (160–200cm) of surgical tubing from a pharmacy. Screw an eye bolt into a door jamb, or into a wall in the garage, anchor the middle of the band to the bolt. Tie knots in the end of the tubes, or make a handle, then pull, using alternating arms or using both arms together. Use your muscles in the same range of movement used in your sport, pulling from a spot directly in front of your shoulders to as far back as you can.

Using dumbbells, bricks or heavy books, bend forwards at the waist, then alternately bring your right and left arm as far back as you can. Alternatively, lie on your back with your arms on the floor behind your head. Holding the dumbbells, bricks or books, bring your arms upwards, until they are vertical over your head.

Another way to develop these muscles is with a partner. Take two lengths of rope or two poles at least 6ft (120cm) long. Face

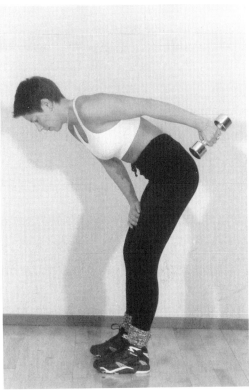

Fig 116

each other, each holding one end of each pole. Both pull back with the right arm, while resisting the other's pull with the left arm; then both pull with the left arm, while resisting with the right arm. Both the

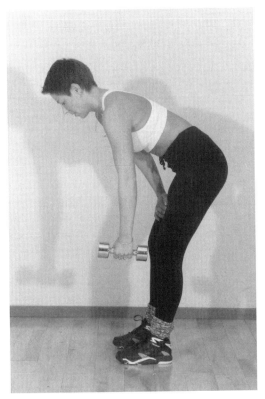

Fig 115

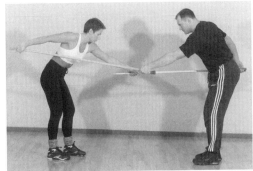

Fig 117

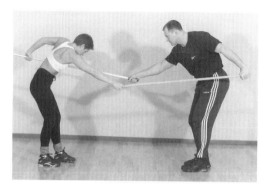

Fig 118

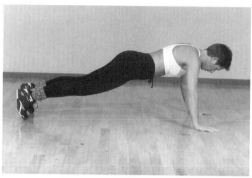

Fig 120

pulling and the resisting are working the 'lats', and one of the three heads of the triceps. While doing this exercise, keep the arms straight.

The Triceps

The triceps ('three heads') straighten (extend) the elbow. One of the three heads crosses the shoulder joint so it works with the lats in pulling the upper arm backwards. All three heads work to straighten the arm at the elbow joint. This is done in the last part of the pulling action.

Use the triceps extension machine at the gym, do triceps extensions on the lat pulldown machine, or lift dumbbells over your

head. Alternatively, you can do push-ups with either your feet or your knees on the floor.

The Front of the Thigh

The muscle at the front of the thigh (the quadriceps) is used in running and kicking. It also helps to avoid knee injuries if it is strong.

In a gym, use the quadriceps machine. Otherwise, exercise with a partner:

1. sit on a table;
2. have your partner place both hands on your ankle and give resistance;
3. straighten your leg.

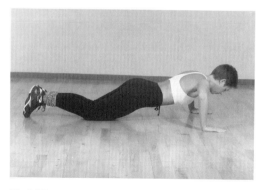

Fig 119

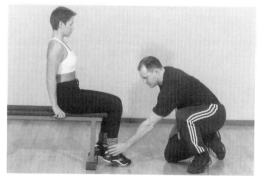

Fig 121

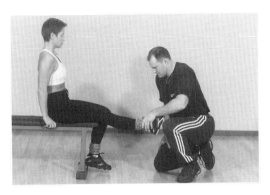

Fig 122

If you don't have a partner, use a rubber band as in the exercise for the upper back.

The Back of the Thigh

The hamstrings at the back of the thigh provide most of the push backwards when running. Use the special machine in the gym, or work with a partner:
1. lie face down on the floor or a table;
2. have your partner push against your ankle as you lift your lower leg from the floor;
3. keep your knee on the floor.

To work the upper part of the rear of the hips, the muscles that do most of the pushing work in your running:

1. lie on a table face down, with your hips on the table, your thighs past the end of the table, and your toes touching the floor;
2. you can use a partner, if you want more strength, or do it alone, if you want more endurance by doing many repetitions;
3. start with one toe touching the floor, then bring the other leg as high as possible;

4. alternate legs. This will look like an exaggerated kicking action for the crawl stroke.

For another partner exercise for hip extension, see the hip flexion exercise.

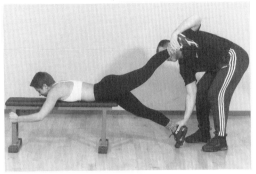

Fig 123

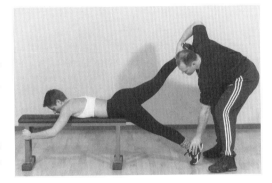

Fig 124

Hip and Knee Extension

This exercise will give you greater force potential from your hips and knees. At the gym, use squat racks or other machines that allow you to extend your legs. At home, do simple three-quarter knee bends (don't bend your knees over 90 degrees).

If you want twice the resistance, do the exercise one leg at a time. To do a one leg

183

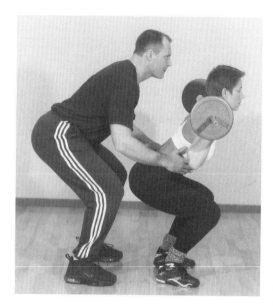

Fig 125

half bend, hold a table top to steady yourself. Using only one leg, bend down 45 to 90 degrees, then return to a standing position. By doing it on only one leg you get the same effect as squatting with two legs while holding a barbell equal to your own weight.

Calf Muscles

The calf muscles (the gastrocnemius and soleus) can be exercised by simply rising up on the toes, then bringing the heels back to the ground. Repeat many times for endurance. If you want more strength, such as for jumping or hill climbing, balance yourself by holding a table or chair

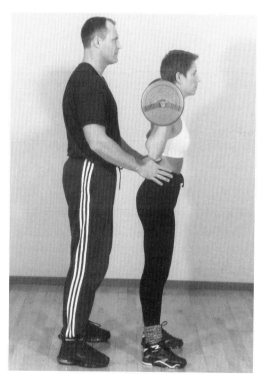

Fig 126

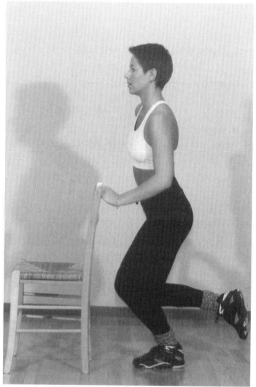

Fig 127

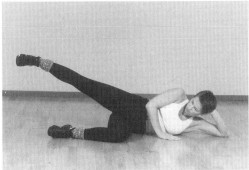

Fig 129

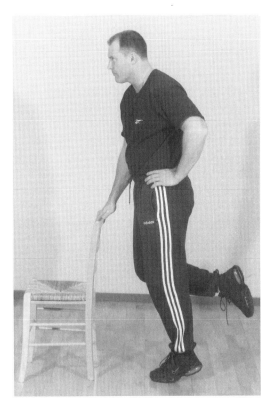

Fig 128

then do the exercise using only one leg at a time – do the right leg until it is exhausted, then the left leg until it is exhausted.

Hip Abductors

The abductors, on the outside of the lower hip, are the muscles that move the legs sideways away from the mid-line of the body. They are very important in helping to maintain balance. When you reach one leg out to the side, such as when 'guarding' in netball or basketball, or moving laterally along the baseline in tennis, you are using the abductors, which stop your motion outwards.

At the gym, use the 'multi-hip' machine, or the low pulley weights with ankle straps. Stand with one side of your body next to the machine and put the ankle strap on the leg farthest from the machine. Lift the leg sideways, keeping it straight.

With a partner, lie on your side. Let your partner put pressure on your knee or ankle, then lift your leg as high as you can. If you have no partner you can do the same exercise alone; you won't get as strong, but you can get just as much endurance. You can also do it yourself by sitting with your knees close to your chest then giving pressure with your hands to the outside of your knees as you bring your knees outwards.

You can also use the rubber bands. Attach one to a low part of a wall, hook your foot into a loop on the end of the band, and lift your leg outwards.

Hip Adductors

The hip adductors are the muscles high on the inside of the thighs, which bring the legs back to the body's middle. The exercises are the reverse of those for the abductors. The adductors are often pulled or strained, so it is wise to keep them in good shape.

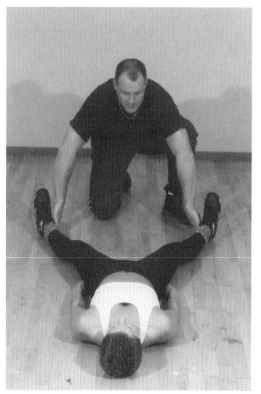

Fig 130

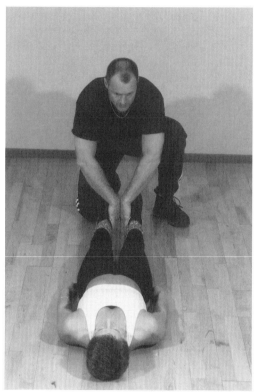

Fig 131

At the gym, use the low pulley station on the machine. Stand sideways to the pulley, 3ft (1 metre) away from the machine. Put the ankle strap on the ankle nearest the machine. Let your leg move outwards (towards the machine) with the weight, then bring it back to the other leg.

With a partner, lie on your back with legs apart. Your partner gives pressure inside your ankles. Bring your legs back together. You can combine the adductor and abductor muscles in this exercise. While lying on your back your partner gives hand pressure on the outside of both ankles; spread your legs against the pressure for the abductors. Your partner then gives you pressure on the inside of your ankles and you bring your legs back

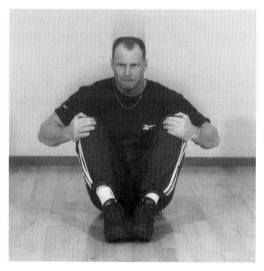

Fig 132

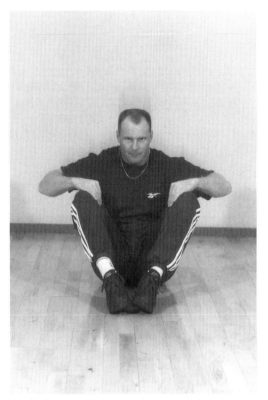

Fig 133

ankles and you bring your legs back together (for the adductors).

Without a partner, sit on the floor with your feet about 12in (20cm) from your hips, and heels together. Spread your knees outwards, then grasp the inside of your knees with your hands. Bring your knees together as you resist the movement with your hands. You will feel the tension inside your upper thighs.

Hip Flexion

Hip flexion exercises help you to bring your leg forwards quickly when running, or to kick downwards in swimming. It can be done on a multi-hip machine or with a partner.

With a partner, lie on your right side. With your left leg back, as if you have just finished a long stride, have your partner put pressure on the front of your ankle, then bring your leg as far forwards as you can. The farther forward you go, the less power you will have, so your partner will need to apply less pressure as you move your leg forwards.

Once the leg is forward, your partner can put pressure on the back of your heel, then you can swing your leg back as far as it will go. This is hip extension.

Thigh Rotation

Thigh rotation develops the muscles that rotate the legs, important in skiing. The action is done high in the hips. Sit on the floor with your legs stretched out. Turn your feet inwards as far as they can go, and hold. Then twist outwards, and hold. It is more effective if a partner can give your feet resistance in each direction.

Lower Back

Lower-back exercises should be more geared to muscular endurance than strength, so you should do many repetitions. Lie on the floor face down; lift your shoulders about 6in (15cm) from the floor, then return to the floor. (Don't go too high with your shoulders, because you don't want to create a 'sway back' in your exercise.) Since the lower back is very often injured or strained, this is the most important exercise you can do for injury prevention.

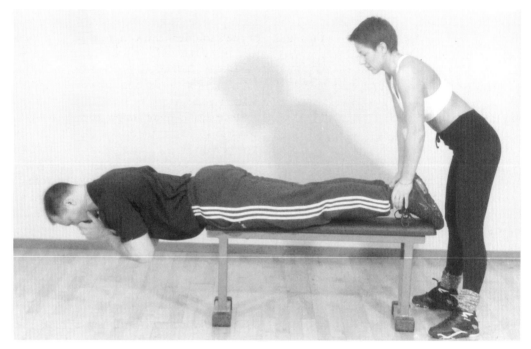

Fig 134

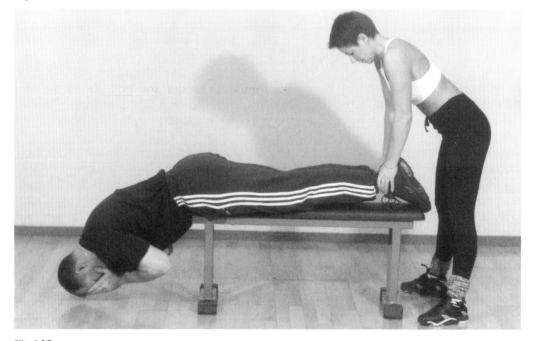

Fig 135

To exercise with a partner, ask the partner to hold your legs. With your hips and legs on a table, bend forwards at the waist to 60 or 90 degrees, then lift your torso back up so that it is in line with your legs and hips. Again, don't arch your back during the exercise.

Repetitions and Weights

The number of repetitions you do and the size of the weights you use depend on your goals. For strength, you should be exhausted in 1 to 3 repetitions. If you are a weight-lifter, a shot putter, or a wrestler you need strength. Skiers or runners, for example, need a certain amount of strength and muscular endurance, and should be doing from 20 to over 100 repetitions.

With a partner, using manual resistance can actually be better than using weights. Unlike weights, your partner can adjust the pressure to make you work to a maximum level on each repetition. Only partners and 'isokinetic' machines have this capability.

Becoming More Flexible

Flexibility comes from stretching the body's different types of connective tissue: that which holds one bone to another (ligaments), that which holds muscles to bones (tendons), and that which holds the individual muscle bundles together. If you are not flexible, you will not have a full range of motion for each joint. When you are too tight you must use excess muscle power just to make a simple movement.

If the connective tissue in the front of your hips is too tight, you won't be able to extend your leg as far backwards when running. If the connective tissue in the front of the shoulders is too tight, you will swim less effectively. Also, if you are not sufficiently flexible, it is easier to sprain (ligament damage) or strain (muscular or tendon damage).

Flexibility is quite simple to achieve. The connective tissue tends to shorten if it is not kept stretched, so most people have lost some flexibility over the years. Stretches should be held for twenty to thirty seconds in order to get the maximum benefits. If you find that you are particularly tight in one area, do the exercise several times a day.

The Toe Touch

This exercise keeps your lower back and the back of your hips and thighs flexible. While most people do it standing, it is more effective to do it sitting on the floor. When you are sitting and stretching forwards, the muscles in the back of your torso and thighs relax, so you can stretch farther. When you are standing, those same muscles remain somewhat tight because they are fighting the gravity that is allowing you to bend downwards.

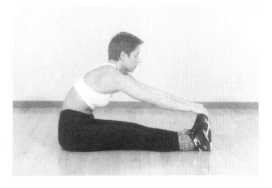

Fig 136

The Leg Straddle

This exercise stretches the tissue of the upper inner thighs, allowing you to spread your legs more easily in a sideways movement. While standing, move your feet sideways, wriggling them farther and farther out each day.

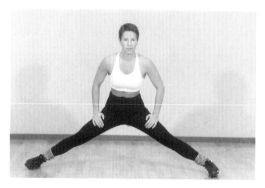

Fig 137

The Splits

This is a forward–backward stretch for the tissue at the front and the rear of the upper thighs. Becoming flexible in these areas makes it easier to do any long striding when running or cross-country skiing. It also makes it easier to kick in soccer or

rugby. Put the right foot forwards and the left back. Keep moving them farther and farther apart. Then put the left leg forwards and the right back, and do the same again.

The Upper Chest and Shoulder Stretch

This exercise is not only good to prevent round shoulders but will also allow you to use a longer poling action in cross-country skiing. With your arms at shoulder level, pull them backwards as far as they will go, and hold the position.

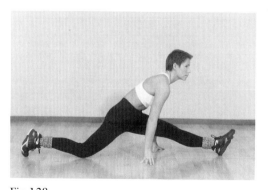

Fig 138

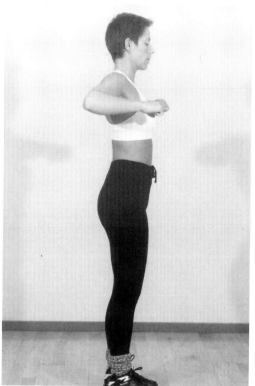

Fig 139

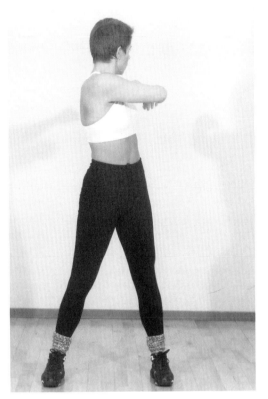

Fig 140

Trunk Twist

This exercise stretches the middle of your torso. You will want to be flexible in this area, especially for soccer, volleyball or basketball. You can stretch from the sitting position or the standing position.

The Front of the Shoulder Stretch

This exercise allows you to push further back with your arms in the poling action of cross-country skiing, or to make an easier recovery stroke in swimming. While standing with your arms at your side, bring both arms directly backwards as far as you can, and hold the position.

Effective conditioning helps your body to be the best tool that it can be for effective athletic movement. It keeps your physiological age reduced, makes you look and feel better, and will certainly reduce your chances of injury.

Information on Vitamins and Minerals

Vitamin	Solubility	RDA Recommended (Minimum) Daily Allowance	Functions	Deficiencies and excesses	Sources
A	Fat soluble stored in body	Men: 5,000 units (RE-retinol equivalents) Women: 4,000 units (800 RE) Toxic level: 10,000 to 50,000 units (2,000 to 10,000 RE) (if all from animal sources)	1. Formation of body tissue 2. Development of mucous secretions in nose, mouth, digestive tract, organs (which show bacterial entry) 3. Development of visual purple in the retina of the eye-which allows one to see in the dark 4. Produces the enamel-producing cells of the teeth 5. Assists normal growth 6. Estrogen synthesis 7. Sperm production	Deficiencies can cause night blindness, damaged intestinal tract, damaged reproductive tract, scaly skin. poor bones, dry mucous membranes, and in children, poor enamel in the teeth. Toxic symptoms (of Retinol): may mimic brain tumour (increased pressure inside the skull), weight loss, irritability, loss of appetite, severe headaches, vomiting, itching, menstrual irregularities, diarrhoea, fatigue, skin lesions, bone and joint pains, loss of hair, liver and spleen enlargement, and insomnia. In children, overdose can stunt growth.	Butter and margarine Whole milk Liver Fish Fortified non-fat milk Fish liver oils Egg yolks
Beta-carotene		As antioxidant 25,000 to 50,000 units (15 to 30 mg)	1. Precurser to vitamin A 2. Antioxidant Reduces cancer risk Reduces heart disease	Deficiency: Increased free oxygen radical activity. Excess: may yellow the skin.	Carrots Broccoli Dark Green or orange fruits or vegetables

Vitamin	Solubility	RDA Recommended (Minimum) Daily Allowance	Functions	Deficiencies and excesses	Sources
B1 (thiamin)	Water soluble	1.5mg (men) 1.2mg (women)	1. Metabolizes carbohydrates 2. Resulting glucose (sugar) nourishes muscles and nerves 3. Aids nerve functioning	Deficiencies can cause: mental depression, moodiness, quarrelsomeness and unco-operativeness, fatigue, irritability, lack of appetite, muscle cramps, constipation, nerve pains (due to degeneration of myelin sheath which covers the nerve), weakness and feeling of heaviness in the legs, beri-beri (a disease in which the muscles atrophy and become paralysed)	Liver Pork Yeast Organ meats Whole grains Bread Wheat germ Peanuts Milk Eggs Soya beans
B2 (riboflavin)	Water soluble	1.8mg (men) 1.4mg (women)	1. Effects rate of growth and Metabolic rate since it is necessary for the cell's use of protein, fat, and carbohydrate 2. Growth 3. Adrenal cortex activity 4. Red blood cell formation	Deficiencies can cause: burning and itching eyes, blurred and dim vision, eyes sensitive to light, inflammation of the lips and tongue, lesions at the edges of the mouth, digestive disturbances, greasy, scaly skin, personality problems	Eggs Liver and other organs Yeast Milk Whole grains Bread Wheat germ Green leafy vegetables
B3 (niacin or nicotinic acid)	Water soluble Limited storage in body	20mg (men) 15mg (women)	1. Similar to riboflavin in metabolizing foods (especially sugars) 2. Maintain normal skin conditions 3. Aids in functioning of the gastro-intestinal tract	Deficiencies can cause: Dermatitis (red, tender skin, becoming scaly and ulcerated), fatigue, sore mouth (tongue), diarrhoea, vomiting, nervous disturbances, mental depression, anorexia, weight loss, headache, backache, mental confusion, irritability, hallucinations, delusions of persecution, pellagra. Large doses can be toxic because it dilates blood vessels. Can cause skin flushing, dizziness, head throbbing, also dryness of skin, itching, brown skin pigmentation, decreased glucose (sugar) tolerance and perhaps a rise in uric acid in the blood	Yeast Liver Wheat bran Peanuts Beans

Vitamin	Solubility	RDA Recommended (Minimum) Daily Allowance	Functions	Deficiencies and excesses	Sources
Pantothenic acid	Water soluble Little storage in body	4–7 mg	1. Carbohydrate, fat and protein metabolism 2. Synthesis of cholesterol and steroid hormones 3. Aids the functioning of the adrenal cortex 4. Aids in choline metabolism	Almost never deficient in human diets. Various animals studies have shown different results from deficiency: rough skin, diarrhoea, anaemia, possible coma convulsions, hair loss, and many other symptoms. But they have not been shown in humans	Liver Organ meats Yeast Wheat bran Legumes Cereals
Biotin	Water soluble	0–3 mg	Metabolism of amino acids, fatty acids and carbohydrates	Deficiencies are extremely rare. Raw egg whites which combine with the biotin in the intestines and make it unavailable and some antibiotics (which kill the biotin-producing organization in the intestines) could cause a deficiency Deficiency would be marked by: dry, scaly skin, grey pallor (skin colour) slight anaemia, muscular pains, weakness, depression and loss of appetite	Manufactured in the intestines Also found in: liver yeast kidney egg yolks
B₆ (pyridoxine)	Water soluble	2.0 mg (men) 2.0 mg (women)	1. Catalyst in protein, fat, and carbohydrate metabolism. A high protein diet increases the need for B-6 2. Converts tryptophan to niacin 3. Assists in nervous system 4. Antibody production	Anaemia, dizziness, nausea, vomiting, irritability, confusion, kidney stones, skin and mucous membrane problems. In infants: irritability, muscle twitching, convulsion. Excesses – impaired sensation in limbs. Unsteady gait.	Usually not necessary to supplement Wheat germ Kidney Liver Ham Organ meats Legumes Peanuts

Vitamin	Solubility	RDA Recommended (Minimum) Daily Allowance	Functions	Deficiencies and excesses	Sources
Folic acid (folacin)		0.2–0.4 mg	1. Aids in maturation of red and white blood cells 2. May assist in the synthesis of nucleic acids 3. DNA synthesis	Blood disorders, anaemia, diarrhoea Deficiencies most likely to occur during pregnancy and lactation	Yeast Liver Egg yolk Green leafy vegetables
B12	Water soluble stored in the body	60 mg (men & women)	1. Controls blood forming defects and nerve involvement in pernicious anaemia 2. Involved in protein, fat, carbohydrates, nucleic acid and folic acid metabolism. 3. Necessary to the normal functioning of cells, especially in the bone marrow, nervous system and intestinal tract	Sore tongue, amenorrhoea, signs of degeneration of the spinal cord, anaemia, heart and stomach trouble, headache, and fatigue	Liver organ meats Oysters Salmon Eggs Beef Milk

Vitamin	Solubility	RDA Recommended (Minimum) Daily Allowance	Functions	Deficiencies and excesses	Sources
C (ascorbic acid)	Water soluble Little body storage	60 mg. 10 mg per day prevents scurvy Recommended as anti-oxidant: 1–1½ g	1. Forms collagen intracellular cement which strengthens cell walls (especially the small blood vessels and capillaries), tooth dentine, cartilage, bones and connective tissue 2. Aids in the absorption of iron 3. Aids in formation of red blood cells in the bone marrow 4. Aids in the metabolism of some amino acids (phenylalanine and tyrosine) 5. May be involved in the synthesis of steroid hormones from cholesterol 6. Any body stress may deplete the vitamin C in the tissues which may increase shock, or bacterial infections 7. Antioxidant	Scurvy results from low vitamin C intake. Minor symptoms of vitamin C deficiency could be: subcutaneous haemorrhages (bleeding below the skin), bleeding from gums, swollen gums Excess of vitamin C can result in kidney stones and diarrhoea, destruction of B_{12}, acidosis	Citrus Fresh fruits Berries Broccoli Tomatoes Green leafy vegetables Baked potatoes Turnips

Vitamin	Solubility	RDA Recommended (Minimum) Daily Allowance	Functions	Deficiencies and excesses	Sources
D	Stored in liver Fat soluble	400 units (10 mcgm) Toxic level: 1,000 to 1,500 units (25 to 38 mcgm)	1. Assists in the development of bones and teeth by aiding calcium to harden 2. Facilitates the absorption of calcium and phosphorus, lack of which can cause muscular cramping 3. Neuromuscular activity	Deficiencies: rickets (children), osteomalacia (women who have had frequent pregnancies and poor diets). Teeth may be more susceptible to caries (cavities), Cramping in muscles if there is a low level of calcium or phosphorus in the blood. Soft bones, bowed legs, poor posture Toxic symptoms: fatigue, weight loss, nausea, vomiting, weakness, headache, kidney damage, kidney stones, hardening of the soft tissue of the heart, blood vessels, lungs, stomach and kidneys. Increases cholesterol level of blood. Makes bones more fragile. High levels in developing foetuses and young children may cause mental retardation or blood vessel malformation (especially a blockage in the aorta – the major artery from the heart)	Exposure to ultraviolet light (sunlight) can give minimum daily requirements by changing one type of cholesterol to vitamin D Milk Fish liver oils Egg yolk Butter Whole milk Non-fat milk (with D) Margarines (with D added)
E (tocopherol)	Fat soluble not stored in body	10 units 10 mg TE (tocopherol equivalents) As an antioxidant: 400 units (TE) 600 units (if over 50 years, 2,500 if heavy exerciser)	1. It is thought to stabilize membranes. 2. May be helpful in stablizing Vitamin A. 3. May be necessary in diets high in polyunsaturated fats. 4. Aids in sythesizing red blood cells. 5. Antioxidant.	No known deficiency symptoms in human adults. Some premature infants apparently do not immediately develop the ability to absorb the vitamin	Synthesized in the intestines. Alpha tocopherol D Alpha tocopherol E better than mixed-tocopherol E. Human milk (cow's milk poor) Margarine Oil salad dressing Cereal germ Green leafy vegetables

Vitamin	Solubility	RDA Recommended (Minimum) Daily Allowance	Functions	Deficiencies and excesses	Sources
K	Fat soluble	Men: 80 mcgm Women: 63 mcgm	Helps in the production of prothrombin (blood clotting agent)	Antibiotics taken orally (which could kill the synthesizing bacteria) or diarrhoea (which could flush out the bacteria) could possibly cause a deficiency. Newborn infants, especially premature babies, often suffer from a deficiency. This may cause excessive bleeding. Toxic symptoms in infants: jaundice, mild anaemia	Synthesized by intestinal bacteria Green leafy vegetables Cabbage Cauliflower. Smaller amounts in: tomatoes, egg yolk, and whole milk

Mineral	Solubility	RDA Recommended (Minimum) Daily Allowance	Functions	Deficiencies and excesses	Sources
Calcium		1,200 mg	Development of strong bones and teeth. Helps muscles contract and relax normally, Utilization of iron. Normal blood clotting. Maintenance of body neutrality. Normal action of heart muscle	Rickets, porous bones, bowed legs, stunted growth, slow clotting of blood, poor tooth formation, tetany	Milk, cheese, mustard, turnip, green, clams, oyster, broccoli, cauliflower, cabbage, molasses, nuts. Small amount in egg, carrot, celery, orange, grapefruit, figs, and bread made with milk
Fluorine		1.5–4 mg	Resistance to dental caries. Deposition of bone calcium. May be involved in iron absorption	Deficiencies: weak teeth and bones, anaemia, impaired growth. At levels of 1.5 to 4 parts per million teeth will be strong, but may be mottled. At levels over 6 ppm teeth and bones may be deformed	Water supply containing 1 ppm. Small amounts in many foods
Iodine		0.15 mg	Constituent of thyroxine which is a regulator of metabolism Synthesis of vitamin A	Enlarged thyroid gland. Low metabolic rate, stunted growth retarded, mental growth	Iodized salt Sea foods Food grown in non-goitrous regions

Mineral	Solubility	RDA Recommended (Minimum) Daily Allowance	Functions	Deficiencies and excesses	Sources
Iron		10 mg (men) 15 mg (women)	Constituent of haemoglobin, which carries oxygen to the tissues Collagen synthesis, antibody production	Nutritional anaemia, pallor, weight loss, fatigue, weakness, retarded growth	Red meats, especially liver, green vegetables, yellow fruits, prunes, raisins, legumes, whole grain and enriched cereals, molasses, egg yolk, potatoes, oysters
Magnesium		350–400 mg (men) 280–300 mg (women)	Activates various enzymes. Assists in breakdown of phosphates and glucose necessary for muscle contractions. Regulates body temperature. Assists in synthesizing protein Tooth enamel stability	Failure to grow, pallor, weakness, irritability of nerves and muscles, irregular heartbeat, heart and kidney damage, convulsions and seizures, delirium, depressions	Soya flour, whole wheat, oatmeal, peas, brown rice, whole corn, beans, nuts, soybeans, spinach, clams
Phosphorus		800–1,200 mg (men & women)	Development of bones and teeth. Multiplication of cells. Activation of some enzymes and vitamins. Maintenance of body neutrality. Participates in carbohydrate metabolism ADP/ATP synthesis acid/base balance DNA/RNA synthesis	Rickets, porous bones, bowed legs, stunted growth, poor tooth formation. Excesses of phosphorus may have same effect on the bones as deficient calcium (osteoporosis porous bones)	Milk, cheese, meat, egg yolk, fish, nuts, whole grain cereals, legumes, Soya flour, whole wheat, oatmeal, peas, brown rice, whole corn, beans

Mineral	Solubility	RDA Recommended (Minimum) Daily Allowance	Functions	Deficiencies and excesses	Sources
Potassium		2.5 grams	Acid-base balance. Carbohydrate metabolism. Conduction of nerve impulses Contraction of muscle fibres. May assist in lowering blood pressure (if consumed in equal proportions as sodium)	Apathy, muscular weakness, poor gastro-intestinal tone, respiratory muscle failure, tachycardia (irregular heartbeat), cardiac arrest (heart stops beating)	Soya beans, cantaloupe, sweet potatoes, avocado, raisins, banana, halibut, sole, baked beans, molasses, ham, mushroom, beef, white potatoes, tomatoes, kale, radishes, prune juice, nuts and seeds, wheat germ, green leafy vegetables, cocoa, vegetable juices, cream of tartar, prunes, figs, apricots, oranges, grapefruit
Selenium		70 mcgm men 55 mcgm women As an antioxidant: up to 100 for heavy exercisers	Antioxidant – may reduce risk of stomach and esophageal cancers	Toxic level: nausea, hair loss, diarrhea, irritability.	Organ meats meats milk fruits (depends on the amount of selenium in the soil)

Mineral	Solubility	RDA Recommended (Minimum) Daily Allowance	Functions	Deficiencies and excesses	Sources
Sodium		1–2 grams (⅕ to ⅖ teaspoon)	Constraint of extra-cellular fluid. Maintenance of body neutrality. Osmotic pressure. Muscle and nerve irritabilty Acid/base balance	Muscle cramps, weakness, headache, nausea, anorexia, vascular collapse Excess may raise blood pressure	Sodium chloride (table salt) Sodium bicarbonate (baking soda) Monosodium glutamate The greatest portion of sodium is provided by table salt and salt used in cooking. Foods high in sodium include: dried beef, ham, canned corned beef, bacon, wheat breads, salted crackers, flaked breakfast cereals, olives, cheese, butter, margarine, sausage, dried fish, canned vegetables, shellfish and salt water fish, raw celery, egg white.
Zinc		15 mg men 12 mg women	Metabolism, formation of nucleic acid Enzyme formation Collagen production, fetal development, enhanced appetite and taste	Impaired growth, sexual development, skin problems	Beef, chicken, fish, beans, whole wheat, cashew nuts

Index